WIRED OUR OWN WAY

Wired Our Own Way

AN ANTHOLOGY OF IRISH AUTISTIC VOICES

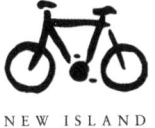

NEW ISLAND

Edited by
NIAMH GARVEY

WIRED OUR OWN WAY
First published in 2025 by
New Island Books
Glenshesk House
10 Richview Office Park
Clonskeagh
Dublin D14 V8C4
Republic of Ireland
newisland.ie

Introduction © Niamh Garvey, 2025
Individual Essays © Individual Authors, 2025

The right of the authors to be identified as the authors of these works has been asserted in accordance with the provisions of the Copyright and Related Rights Act, 2000.

Print ISBN: 978-1-83594-005-1
eBook ISBN: 978-1-83594-006-8
Audiobook ISBN: 978-1-83594-007-5

All rights reserved. The material in this publication is protected by copyright law. Except as may be permitted by law, no part of the material may be reproduced (including by storage in a retrieval system) or transmitted in any form or by any means; adapted; rented or lent without the written permission of the copyright owners.

British Library Cataloguing in Publication Data. A CIP catalogue record for this book is available from the British Library.

Product safety queries can be addressed to New Island Books at the above postal address or at info@newisland.ie.

Set in 12 on 15pt in Bembo
Typeset by JVR Creative India
Edited by Niamh Garvey
Cover design by Niall McCormack, hitone.ie
Printed by SprintBooks, Dublin, Ireland

New Island received financial assistance from The Arts Council (An Comhairle Ealaíon), Dublin, Ireland.

New Island Books is a member of Publishing Ireland.

10 9 8 7 6 5 4 3

Contents

Introduction   1

This Magical Life
Jen Wallace   13

Karma Chameleon
Liam Coulson   19

Righting the Applecart: Of Perfectionism, Friendship and Self-Compassion
Nuala O'Connor   25

Autistic at Seventy
Jane Cadman   37

Growing
Eric Crowley   45

Discovering Autism
James McClean   53

Thirteen
Róisín Riley   59

Poetic Justice
Fiacre Ryan   67

Key Words
Fiacre Ryan   68

How Not to Write a Musical Composition
Justin Bakker   75

Life as a Second Language
Naoise Dolan   83

Makeshift Oasis
Colm Brady   95

The Canary
    Freya von Noorden Pierce   103
Co-Regulating Chaos
    Anonymous   109
The Tin Man's Heart
    Jennifer Poyntz   117
'I don't have a defective version of what you've got'
    Stefanie Preissner   125
Rizz 'Em with the 'Tism
    Chandrika Narayanan-Mohan   133
I'm So Burnt Out I Can Smell the Smoke
    Emil E. Osiński   143
Sharing Spaces
    Stuart Neilson   151
A Tale of Two Lockdowns
    Caoimhe O'Gorman   159
My Path to Advocacy
    Adam Harris   167
Radical Love
    Priyangee Guha   179
Dordán (Drone)
    Mike McGrath-Bryan   185
Ticklish Brain
    Aisling Walsh   193
The Magic of Books
    Cliona Kelliher   201

Timeline of Autism Diagnosis: An Overview   207
A Note on Language around Autism   210
Glossary   211
Acknowledgements   215

Introduction
by Niamh Garvey

To be open and honest about being autistic requires a large dollop of courage. When I tell people that I am autistic, it can feel like an X-ray scanner is turned upon me, while the person searches for signs of autism in me – do I 'look' autistic, do I speak differently, do I move my body in repetitive ways, and do I match the label of 'autism' at all? Many people do not understand what being autistic actually means, and subconsciously carry outdated assumptions about what an autistic person should or shouldn't look like, or what they can or cannot do. But autism does not have a 'look', just as non-autistic people do not all look the same. This anthology of essays shows how radically different the lived experiences of autism can be.

When writing an essay, it is up to the writer to disclose what they want the reader to know about themselves. Each writer began with the same empty page, free to express themselves without being stereotyped according to their ability to speak or not speak, their cultural background, skin colour, sexuality and whether or not they have visibly obvious autistic traits such as poor eye contact or repetitive body movements. In turn, the reader is freed from the clutter of assumptions and can approach each essay with unveiled eyes. The reader and the autistic writer therefore begin on equal footing, which can be quite the opposite of the lived experience of many autistic people when it comes to first impressions.

The form of the essay also frees people who don't fit into stereotypical presentations of autism, many of whom have had their autism repeatedly disbelieved. In particular, autistic women can experience scepticism when we tell someone that we are autistic, which is shown in the essay by Jennifer Poyntz, whose doctor told her, '*You just don't really fit the bill, if you know what I mean.*'

Part of the reason that people often don't believe those of us who disclose our autism is that public perception has yet to catch on that being autistic is not something to be afraid of, nor ashamed of. As Eric Crowley writes, '*I think people still see us as a hindrance, or something to look after.*' When people think that to be autistic is to be something 'less', it contributes to stigmatisation that has real-life consequences, as Priyangee Guha explains: '*Talking about being autistic is strongly detrimental to me in inconceivable ways. I may be refused employment, or medical treatment, or legal rights, or dates, or friendships.*'

All writers were given the choice of writing anonymously, using a pen name, or using their actual name. This might seem like an unusual thing to offer writers in an anthology, but it felt like a necessary step to take as editor; an offer of a shield against the vulnerable position we are placed in when we speak about our autism.

One in twenty-seven school children in Ireland are now formally diagnosed as autistic (no doubt with many more unidentified or awaiting assessment), which sensationalist media sometimes labels as an epidemic, but I celebrate as a sign of increased understanding and thus identification of autism. When I was a child in the eighties and nineties, it was rare to get a diagnosis of autism. Even though my behaviours and language development necessitated me being seen by a developmental paediatrician, a speech and language therapist and a psychologist, no one ever suggested that I was autistic. On the other hand, many people who *were* diagnosed as children in the eighties and nineties experienced 'treatments', therapies and methods of education that have now been recognised as cruel and traumatising – the focus lay on extinguishing autistic behaviour and trying to make autistic children act and appear more 'normal'.

The label of 'autism' is a relatively new diagnosis, having only become an official stand-alone diagnosis in the 1980s, despite autism being an age-old neurotype. There's copious evidence of autism throughout history, right back to many of the Irish children accused of being changelings. Throughout the early to mid-1900s, autistic people who *did* get a diagnosis were labelled with either schizophrenia or mental retardation. In the 1960s, the label of 'autism' came into play, but it was classified as a form of schizophrenia. In her essay 'Autistic at Seventy' Jane Cadman explains that '*Autism did not exist when I was a child, unless it was extreme male autism.*'

During this time, Irish autistic people who had higher support needs tended to be institutionalised, which I believe is one of the reasons I so often hear people say, 'Sure there were no autistic people back in my day.' Those who were *not* hidden away in institutions tended to collect alternative labels, as shown in multiple essays, such as Liam Coulson recounting being called a '*retard*', '*thick*' and '*strange*', and Colm Brady being called '*weird*'.

Nowadays, many adults in Ireland are finally discovering their *real* label of 'autism' and finding validation in that. When I was getting assessed for autism at the age of thirty-four, many people asked me why I would seek out being labelled as 'autistic'. Their confusion was laced with the undertone that to be 'autistic' is to be something undesirable, and that if I could 'pass' without the label, then I should. I explained that if my brain was wired differently, then the label of 'autism' would not change my wiring, but at least I would understand how my mind worked, and what actions I could take to make life easier. Chandrika Narayanan-Mohan explains that '*with more information about how my brain works, the anxieties and barriers have started to fall away*'.

Contrary to an increasingly popular accusation in the media, getting diagnosed as autistic is not a 'lifestyle choice'; it is simply a matter of clarifying one's identity. Eighteen-year-old writer Róisín Riley succinctly sums this up: '*For just one person to recognise who I was, to suggest that I was the autistic person that I didn't even know I was, it changed everything ... To understand that I don't need to be changed, I need to be recognised.*'

Before people learn that they are autistic, they often feel like a flawed human being, as they don't understand their challenges and differences. Aisling Walsh writes that before her diagnosis, '*I spent most of my adult life believing I was broken.*' Autism identification allows people to become comfortable with themselves and their differences, as Nuala O'Connor explains in her essay: '*In the last few years (since autism diagnosis) – after a lifetime of befuddlement – I've found I belong right here in this body, and in this mind, uncomfortable and challenging as that can be.*'

Many of us autistic people learn to mask our differences from a young age, moulding ourselves on how other people behave, as Caoimhe O'Gorman experienced: *'My friends and my teachers never saw me melt down; something I'd purposely hidden because I was ashamed. I didn't know they were autistic meltdowns for a long time and instead thought I was just too sensitive.'*

This masking survival tactic is one of many reasons that has been shown in research to contribute to the significantly higher rates of depression and anxiety amongst autistic people. A number of the essays submitted showed a common experience of adults not finding out they were autistic until they accessed mental health services (often in crisis), as mentioned in the essays by Stuart Neilson and Róisín Riley. On the other hand, many writers flagged their suspicions that they were autistic with health professionals, including psychiatrists, only to be told they were not autistic and refused access to an autism assessment. I couldn't include all the essays that showed this type of gaslighting as there were too many, but one I did include is that by Jane Cadman, who missed out on diagnosis until she was sixty-nine.

A frequent route to adult autism identification is when a child is diagnosed as autistic, and the parent realises that they have multiple autistic traits themselves, which is what happened for Irish professional footballer James McClean.

Media representation is another increasingly common route to people realising they are autistic, such as author Nuala O'Connor's epiphany when listening to a radio interview of a late-diagnosed autistic woman. One high-profile woman whose media presence has helped many Irish people recognise autism in themselves is Stefanie Preissner, who speaks openly about her autism through multiple media and social media platforms. I was delighted she agreed to let me include one of her essays on her own late diagnosis, which was previously published in the *Irish Independent*.

Autistic people speaking up about their autism is having a diagnosis-domino affect around the world. Technology is playing a pivotal role in this, both through empowering people to communicate and by connecting autistic people with each other.

Fiacre Ryan's essay shows how his inability to speak meant that he had no method with which to communicate until he began to use AAC (augmentative and assistive technology) aged eleven, beginning with pointing at letters on a board, and now using both a letterboard and a tablet to communicate. Learning how to use an alternative communication method to spoken language led him to becoming the first non-speaking autistic person to do the Junior Cert in Ireland, then the Leaving Cert, and he is now a published writer, poet and university student.

Adam Harris's essay shows how the internet has played a vital role in bringing autistic people together: one blog post in which he shared his frustration around communicating with other people led to him connecting with other autistic people, and ultimately to him setting up Ireland's national autism charity, AsIAm.

A concept that I myself learnt about through conversations with other autistic people online was 'autistic joy'. We autistic people feel our emotions intensely, which can be a challenge when it is an uncomfortable emotion, but can be euphoric when it concerns joy. Multiple essays show different examples of this intense joy, often reached through our special interests. Again, they demonstrate just how vastly different we all are in our personalities and passions, from Cliona Kelliher's soul-strong love of books to Jen Wallace's deep and joyful connection with nature.

Music comes up more than once as a source of autistic joy, from the beloved drone of music that bookmarks Mike McGrath-Bryan's life to the magnetic pull of music-based special interests for Justin Bakker.

Our determination and hyperfixation with special interests can lead us to become highly skilled at things we love, which is shown in the essay by footballer James McClean: '*I became obsessed with training and improving. I looked at the tiny details of what I was doing, and how I could get better and how I could continue to stay on the top of my game.*'

When life's obstacles stop us engaging in our special interests, it not only reduces our episodes of autistic joy, but it tampers with our ability to juggle the demands of being an adult, as shown in the anonymously written essay on parenting as an autistic adult, 'Co-regulating Chaos'.

Stumbling blocks to coping with life's challenges – such as language and communication mismatches, as explored in Naoise Dolan's essay – are raised in many of the essays. Probably the most common blockade that crops up is environmental sensory triggers. Stuart Neilson writes how the sensory elements (noise, light, visual order, and so on.) affect more than just the ambience of a place for autistic people; they can be the difference of whether an environment allows us to interact with other people or get anything done.

Emil Elliot Osiński writes, '*Being autistic shouldn't stop me from being able to function in society*', and yet he fears losing his job if he shows how stressed he truly is at work, particularly from sensory triggers. Irish autistic people have a legal right to reasonable accommodations that facilitate us to work for an employer (under the Employment Equality Act 1998 and 2015) but if we are afraid to disclose our autism for fear of stigma, or failing a job interview, then how can we claim these rights?

I didn't want this book to only show one Irish perspective of autism, and certainly didn't want to only show the stereotypical white, male computer/science genius that we see so often in the media. There is no universal experience of being autistic, so I wanted to ensure that this book represented autistic people from as diverse a range of backgrounds as possible. The contributors range in age from eighteen to mid-seventies, with as equal a gender balance as I could achieve. Some are established, experienced writers, and some have never written an essay before.

One way that I ensured that the essays came from as wide a range of people as possible was that I offered help and accommodations to those who needed or wanted them. I volunteered assistance with transcription, as well as offering individualised essay-writing support: this included editorial assistance for turning ideas into essays, or using a question-and-answers structure instead of the more typical essay-type format. Other accommodations I offered, especially to the writers who are AuDHD (autistic and ADHD), were providing multiple shorter deadlines for essay progression (instead of one daunting final deadline), and 'body doubling', which is a practice of working alongside a person to help them to stay focused.

There are certain cohorts of people in Irish society who are more likely to be autistic, so I specifically aimed to include writers from these groups. For example, autistic people are 3–3.5 times more likely to be gay or bisexual (University of Cambridge, 2024), and over 30 per cent of people presenting to the National Gender Services in Ireland are autistic or neurodivergent (NGS, 2024). There are therefore a number of LGBTQIA+ contributors.

I also sought out essays by people with different cultures within Irish society. A particularly interesting perspective is brought by writers who originally came from different countries, who got to experience Irish culture through a fresh lens compared to those of us who were born and raised in Ireland. This highlights aspects of Irish life that alter one's autistic experience, with Priyangee Guha pointing out, for example, that, '*In Ireland, people rarely say what they mean, or mean what they say.*' In contrast to this, Naoise Dolan writes how living outside of Ireland and speaking other languages can change the way people perceive her autistic social differences: '*Nobody has ever given me as hard a time for my social mistakes in foreign languages as they do for the ones I make in English.*'

I tried to get an essay by an Irish autistic Traveller, as I feel the autistic Traveller voice is an under-represented one in Ireland, and one I would personally love to learn more about. Unfortunately, despite reaching out to a number of organisations and people from the Travelling community, I was unable to find a contributor.

There is often media coverage of late-diagnosed autistic adults, and a number of the essay writers fall into this category. It was important to me that the collection also included autistic people who are not typically given the same public platform, such as those diagnosed as children, and non-speaking autistic adults. I also tried to find more contributors with a co-occurring intellectual disability, mindful that some people with an intellectual disability would be able to write an essay independently, while others would need assistance, and some would be unable to engage in writing an essay at all.

In order to reach out to these under-represented cohorts, I contacted AsIAm, adult learning centres, autistic adult support services, university disability services and social media groups. Although the book does include a small number of essays by people from these cohorts, I would have liked more.

Between 20 and 30 per cent of autistic people cannot speak or have very minimal speech, and they are probably the biggest cohort of autistic adults who bear the brunt of incorrect assumptions. Those who are unable to communicate via the spoken word are often assumed to be unable to think, unable to hear, and unable to take offence if people speak about them in their presence. As Fiacre Ryan, a non-speaking man, writes, '*Some people were reluctant to see past my autistic behaviours and accept that I was intelligent enough to spell words and formulate sentences.*' Non-speaking autistic adults are rarely interviewed on radio and television, even though many of them can communicate via assistive technology or could write/type out answers in advance. The essay form can therefore be a powerful route for non-speaking people to change perceptions.

The autistic writers of this anthology have opened their hearts and shared their stories, showing that we are wired our own way, and we are OK with that. Freya von Noorden Pierce writes, '*The world may not be made for us, but you can make it work for you. In fact, demand that it does.*' Unfortunately, a demand is of no use if it is ignored; we also need individual people, as well as society as a whole, to listen to our voices and allow our individual strengths to shine.

References:
NGS (2004) hse.ie/eng/about/personalpq/pq/2024-pq-responses/february-2024/pq-9431-24-patrick-costello.pdf

University of Cambridge (2024) 'Autistic Individuals are more likely to be LGBTQ+' Available at: cam.ac.uk/research/news/autistic-individuals-are-more-likely-to-be-lgbtq

Jen Wallace is a writer of prose and poetry, a children's author, facilitator and nature guide. She runs creativity and nature connection workshops for all ages. *Dinosaur Pie*, her book for children, is published by Little Island Books. **jenwallacecreates.ie**

This Magical Life

I am made for dappled shade, sea breezes and birdsong, not the relentlessness of modern indoor environments. Artificial lights, synthetic smells and industrial noises set me on alert and cause me distress. The antidote is a quiet outdoor spot, somewhere I feel safe, with plenty of wildness. Away from the distraction of the internet and the never-ending laundry, everything slows down and becomes more manageable and I feel at home in myself.

I didn't know I was autistic until well into adulthood. I had no words for the levels of overwhelm, frustration and otherness I felt as a young person. But I have always been able to regulate and exist happily in wild places. I have lived on sparsely inhabited islands, spent months at sea teaching sailing and become a nature guide and herbalist.

I grew up in a small harbour village and across the road from my home was the entrance to an old, wooded estate. It was populated with ancient oaks, hollowed-out beech trees and chestnut trees that dangled generations of children from rough swings. Much of my childhood was spent damming streams, building camps from fallen branches and having what I considered epic adventures in the woods.

My dad's love language was time together in the outdoors. He had my siblings and I in boats from when we could barely see over the gunwales. We fished for mackerel, learnt to row and explored hidden corners of Cork harbour. I raced sailing dinghies with him from about ten years of age. Right through my struggling teens, he would haul me out of bed on the weekends to get me on the water. In winter, it was woodland walks, which later evolved into hillwalking trips. We'd take to the road every Sunday to go walk the Reeks or the Galtees, Mangerton or the Paps.

There was something about being in the hills that let my mind unfold with the landscape and then narrowed my focus to the path ahead, the next step. I believe I walked my way out of the knots in my own head on those days. One of my most cherished memories is of sitting on the summit of Knockmealdown, the bare brown mountain, eating a packed lunch with my dad and saying very little but together drinking in the view all the way to the sea.

After years of working hard to fit in, I hit complete burnout in college and went into a steep depressive spiral. I quit my English degree as I lost my ability to function in the world. I was still unaware of my neurodivergence, and psychiatric intervention was less than helpful. I struggled to understand what was going on, why I could not cope, why everything seemed so hard. My wonderful parents encouraged me to train and work as a water sports instructor. Being on the water, in the elements, challenged, focused and kept me going through some very tricky years. The sea cleared my head and helped my nervous system regulate enough for me to stay in some sort of balance. I still feel as if I am of the sea. It is my element. I crave the sea when I am inland. It is by the sea that I am now rearing my own family.

When my children were small, they were often reluctant to nap anywhere except the car. As I endlessly drove the back roads near our coastal village I began to take notice of the trees on the roadside. I saw the blackthorn come into bloom in spring, followed by the hawthorn. I needed more information, and so my nature book habit started. I soon began to recognise the shapes of ash and alder, willow and oak. The hedgerows were calling for my attention.

I did a two-year course in herbal and botanical medicine. I experienced connecting with the plants as one living creature to another and it brought me joy and peace to come into closer relationship with the green life all around me. Identifying plants and learning their traditional uses became a strong focus for a few years. The intensity of my interest has now mellowed into an easy relationship. I don't garden as such anymore and we have let a lot of our patch grow wild, with space for both the humans and the other beings we share this place with. The robin also owns here, he is not shy about proclaiming it. There are hedgehogs, frogs, shrews, all kinds of insects who call this home. As the garden rewilds, I find I am rewilding too, healing old institutional wounds, learning my own needs and boundaries and leaning into moving gently through this magical life.

Learning about wildlife keeps my autistic brain happily busy. I love to memorise the names of things and gain deep satisfaction from wandering along hedgerows acknowledging the plants I recognise and looking up those I don't. My phone is accumulating identification apps and our home is ridiculously full of books: sea life, trees, mushrooms, insects, birds, geology, weather.

I love how the names of clouds feel cloudlike in my mouth. Cumulus. Cirrus. Cumulonimbus. I know what weather different cloud types and movements indicate. I can tell where south is by the way the trees grow and can predict tides from the phase of the moon. I want to learn more about stars and rocks, about mycelium and natural navigation. These things are far more real to me than fashion and social media.

This human world of industry and busyness, of bright lights and dense traffic, is often uncomfortable for those of us with heightened sensory and nervous systems. Shopping centres can reduce me to a shaking, wordless shell but in the woods I am truly alive, by the sea I can breathe. When I see friends, we meet for a walk or a swim. It is so much easier to be with people outdoors. Conversation flows as we move through landscapes and here the silences are not awkward.

When my anxiety is high, there are times that I just can't go outside. Going for a walk may mean unexpected encounters with humans, and sometimes I don't feel safe to walk by myself. These times I will connect by looking out the window, having a cup of nettle tea or by doing grounding and centring activities that calm my body and mind. Like all wild beings, sometimes I just need to hide away in my burrow.

My heightened sensory system is also a wonderful tool, I am learning to tune my ears to birdsong. I have an app that helps me identify calls and over the last few years I have begun to recognise more of my avian friends. Just as the hedgerows went from being walls of green to a rich diverse community, so now the web of bird sounds is becoming familiar to me and I am picking out individual threads. The endless chattering outside my window is the house sparrows, or spodgies as my dad calls them, the strident 'chee chur' is a great tit and I can recognise when a predator is near by the calls of the rooks. My ears now seek out birdsong and my eyes are drawn skywards.

I like to imagine the birds are writing in the sky, like drifts of sheet music, and I watch trying to decipher the code. I imagine that for millennia, until quite recently, the sky would be filled with huge flocks, that the sound of wingbeats would have been a constant in my ancestors' day.

Some days I am deeply aware of the emptiness of the sky and the vast expanses between trees, how they stretch their roots and canopies looking for community. Living in connection with the natural world also means feeling pain at the destruction and thoughtless demolition that is going on all around us. I don't think it is possible to feel the wonder without also acknowledging the hurt. It can be overwhelming to live in these times and be in awareness of the interconnectedness of every being. For me, the key to coping has been to balance the grief with a deep sense of gratitude. I seek out things to be grateful for and find there is an abundance, and I take action to protect our wild kin in ways I find meaningful.

I feel like an ancient being, finely tuned to feel safe in a harmonious natural environment. No wonder I struggle with human industrial scale discord. There is a deep wisdom here, maybe even a map, of sorts. When I honour the part of me that smiles at dandelions thriving in impossible places, breathes deeply at the smell of earth after rain and excitedly watches every summer for the swallows, then I am at home. At home in myself, at home in this world, at home in this magical life.

Liam Coulson is an autistic writer of tales of the unusual and macabre. He is a graduate of the writing and literature programme at Sligo ATU. Liam lives in the Ox mountains in County Sligo with his Yorkshire terrier, Captain.

Karma Chameleon

Patterns, sequences, I notice them all the time, especially within the senses. They take me back to moments frozen in time. Even today as I wash dishes, with the radio playing a song that once I was mad about.

Suddenly, I am five years old again. It is my birthday, and the year is 1984. I know this because Boy George is singing my favourite song from the tinny radio in Father's van. He hated that I loved Boy George so much. But today he didn't seem to mind me turning 'Karma Chameleon' way up. Back then, I had to hide my fascination with the singer's long, colourful hair and immaculately made-up face.

I had always thought it silly that boys couldn't wear make-up; even sillier was the fact that girls were not allowed to wear trousers. I can still see them, shivering in the playground in skirts and lacy white ankle socks.

There is a discomfort in these memories, I can tell because I have digressed to yet another. I do this all the time, but ironically the digressions always seem to lead to ever deeper levels of distress. It is around this time that I also remember sitting in front of the three-way mirror upon Mother's dressing table. With her cherry bomb lipstick, I carefully painted my pouting lips, her peach negligee hanging off my tiny limbs. Her clip-on earrings catching the light as I tilted my head side to side.

I hadn't heard him open the door, but how could I forget that look of horror on Father's face, as his joined mine in the mirror.

Poof, queer. That's what they used to say. These names hurt much more than when they called me 'retard', because I didn't really know what retard meant. I knew I was thick; I had been told so often that I could live with that. But being a poof and a queer, even before you knew you were one yourself, was just too much to comprehend.

That was why he was taking me to school that day. My brothers wouldn't walk with me anymore, because the other kids might hate them, the way they hated me.

The scent of linseed oil fills my nostrils out of nowhere. Father's van always stank of it. It was in the putty he would put into cracks along window frames before he painted them. A bland smell; I hate bland smells, they make me sick. Vanilla is a bland smell, cinnamon is not, neither is mixed spice. Garlic isn't a bland smell, but still it makes me sick, in an oily kind of a way. Which doesn't make sense really and I hate it when things don't make sense. They must, otherwise I keep picking at them until they do.

I can still see that day so clearly: a huge bag of Liquorice Allsorts in my lap to share with my class. But I didn't have a single friend. No one liked that I rocked back and forth. Everybody was always telling me to stop. But why would you stop something that made you feel better?

I did want to fit in, honestly, I did.

But I knew I was too strange, even Mother told me so. A particular sentence picked out in bold from my school report corroborated this insight: 'Liam takes great delight in irritating other children.' I didn't know I was until then. Why didn't they just tell me? That was why I liked pretend people in books much better. I found them less pretend than real people, who never said what they meant.

I remember the nausea, how it would intensify after we passed by the big building that looked like a pirate ship. It was something to do with telephones, but the satellites were sails, and the antenna was a Gorgon figurehead strapped to its bow.

I can feel that tightness in my stomach now, thinking about it. So often, that I find myself mentally back at those school gates, knowing I would not know how to act. The build-up to every event or social interaction feels like I have just passed the big building that looks like a pirate ship.

I watch, powerless to do anything, as Father's van disappears around the corner in my mind's eye. Black exhaust fumes are all that remain, but I can see that small me, bewildered as to how he got there. He doesn't even recall getting out of the van, but there he was, nonetheless.

School always seemed less scary on a dull day, but that day was impossibly bright and shiny. I watch him kick stones across the playground, the classroom door looming ever closer. There are children everywhere. Conversations and shouts spiralling upwards and around, filling him with silent screams.

I watch as my hands close around his tiny ears, my bag of Liquorice Allsorts now just a kaleidoscope of colour as they fall to the ground.

Then I find myself back in my kitchen, light streaming through half-cleaned windows, while I try to make sense of what happened to me. The reason as to why I spend hours on the bed each evening after work, the hairdryer droning on in the background. The only thing which can ground me, a noise that I can be certain of.

I might be able to think about eating later. But by then, supper would consist of anything I could throw into the microwave.

I have to keep reminding myself that, despite my inadequacies, I have managed to get a mortgage. Yet still, many times throughout the day I find myself lost, staring into the sink as I do now. Musing amongst my dirty dishes, wondering how I can begin to wash them up.

When I'm like this, I just want everything to stop, this rush towards nowhere. This endless discomfort with my environment, constantly I seek to make it cease. But out of this impetuousness – one of the things I hate most about myself – came the one thing that saved me.

I tell myself the story of my life over and over, so I can remind myself that I am here, that I am OK.

But I could never be OK, not until I had bought my small cottage in the Ox mountains in County Sligo. It was where mother came from, and a place we had returned to often when we had been a family.

But the real draw for me was that I was able to afford a detached home, modest as it was. I knew I wouldn't need to suffer anyone's noise again. I had only been able to afford a terraced house back in the UK. My hearing was so acute that I could hear my neighbours flushing toilets and climbing stairs. Their noise was a constant intrusion, as if they were coming into my space all the time, uninvited.

This had all stopped now and that suited me just fine. The environment seemed congenial to my love of writing stories, so I decided that I would try and make something of this. I enrolled on a degree course in writing and literature and as part of that enrolment I did some screening that was recommended. It became apparent that I was dyslexic, and it was at this point that I happened to mention how I was often overloaded by lights, noise and smells. How they had such an impact on me that I simply stopped functioning. As it happened, the disability office was running workshops on sensory processing, so I went along.

The facilitators often talked about autism; the symptoms of which seemed so relevant to me. But it was not until the final workshop that I managed to find the courage to ask if there was any point in me investigating this angle further. I was really surprised by their reaction, 'Oh yes, we definitely think you should.'

I was glad I did. After my diagnosis, it was as if suddenly everything made sense. I didn't stop berating myself straight away, that takes time, and sometimes I still hear that inner critic telling me I'm a horrible, useless person who gets everything wrong.

But I don't have to think this way anymore. For I am not any of these things, I am autistic. It's my environment that is wrong, not me. If my environment suited me, I would still be autistic, but it would not affect me the way it does.

At least now I know what to do to help myself, and the answer does not lie in trying to fit in. I don't fit and I won't, no matter how hard I try.

But for the first time in my life, I know that I don't need to.

Nuala O'Connor is a writer and late-diagnosed autistic. Her sixth novel, *Seaborne*, about Irish-born pirate Anne Bonny, was published in 2024 by New Island. She lives in Galway with her family.

Righting the Applecart

Of Perfectionism, Friendship and Self-Compassion

I have always wondered why I am hysterical about time. My whole life has been about tick-tock, Germanic efficiency. I like to have cushions of minutes (or hours or days) wedging up either side of an appointment – I arrive not just timely but early. I feel irritable when I'm not at my writing desk by 9 a.m. I clock-watch, watch-watch, phone-watch. I protect my precious minutes fiercely, and dislike schedule changes, disruption, and/or unexpected events. Nonchalance and flexibility are not concepts I have traditionally embraced. People who are wishy-washy about specifics irritate me. When I was younger, unpunctual potential boyfriends were given black marks; friends who ran late got frost-face on arrival. And yet I'm married to a man whose middle name could be vague; he's goosey about start times, firm details, and clear action. He grew up in a bendy, accommodating family culture, one of 'turn up whenever', whereas I did not.

Clearly this protection of my time is about control and, if I want to be kinder to myself, about getting the best use out of every minute of my life. In my world, there is a time to write, a time to eat, a time to relax; days are sectioned into slots and The Thing must happen within its allotted portion. Otherwise, my cart of balance – and therefore my sanity – gets rakish, and there's a danger that all my apples will end up on the ground, along with my marbles. Do I want an appley-marbley floor? I do not, because this cart-tip can manifest as high anxiety, seething anger, bodily distress, shouting, crying and, often, shame and shutdown, meaning my body and mind go numb, and I need to retreat entirely to recover.

As a child, if my day or plans were upset, I became an all-roaring, all-door-slamming strop; I snarled, swore, hid myself away. Paradoxically – when things were smooth – I was a quiet loner. My outbursts, and the distress they caused me, felt out of control and embarrassing. After a flare-up, I was an immoveable rag doll. I was written off as a brat; a 'falutherin' virago' (my ma); a house devil, street angel (also my ma); I was christened The Little Curser by our neighbour. My tantrums were seen as wilful but, for me, they were a sudden, frantic possession that left me wrung out and cowed. That they continued into adulthood felt doubly shameful; clearly, I really was the bad, brattish person I was told I was.

All my life, my rigidity around time and detail has caused me – and others – tension and misunderstanding; there have been stand-offs and cleavings, fights and meltdowns. I never knew why strict schedules were so crucial to me, why I became irrationally upset over seemingly minor things like flight delays, or guests arriving an hour late. Why could I not relax and – like most others – go with the flow? Because I couldn't. It was that simple. My thinking went, *If X is supposed to happen* now, *why in God's name isn't it happening?!*

Getting a diagnosis of autism in my early fifties has brought clarity around my time-hysteria, and so much else.

I'm what is known as an AuDHDer – an autistic person with ADHD – which causes its own complications, because there are competing actions and desires within my brain. For example, I want things organised, but I struggle with avoidance; I love attending creative performances, but I find it tricky to concentrate and sit still for large chunks of time; I adore routine and clear parameters, but I also crave novelty and new experiences; I have monotropic tendencies, meaning I prefer to go down a tunnel of interest and remain there until the next sparkly tunnel captures my attention.

Because of all this, my type of brain often adopts perfectionism and control as coping mechanisms. Difficulty in relying on working memory makes it necessary for me to cordon things into patterns and slots, so that they can be achieved. If I can make things run 'perfectly' – to a set timetable – my applecart will stay full and balanced and trundle along nicely.

Unfortunately, when things falter or change, I get upset and my thinking becomes intensely self-critical, because having illogically high standards for yourself, and all about you, is problematic. The world doesn't like perfection and rigidity, it's fluid, bouncy and rutted, so this desire to make everything predictable often backfires, leaving people like me discombobulated, lying on the ground in a sea of apples, in pain and clanging internally, unable to right themselves.

My autism diagnosis, though, has meant that *this* era of my life – my fifties – feels fresh and hopeful, in ways my younger years often were not. I wasn't always a hopeless person, but various events and stumbles left me in repeated episodes of depression where I lost hope. Perfectionism does not result in optimal outcomes, it turns out. I couldn't control the secondary infertility I suffered, for example – my body was deficient despite all my efforts. Chronic illness struck me, though I made mostly healthy life choices. And I couldn't seem to sustain friendships because social situations overwhelmed me, meaning I kept to myself, then felt lonely and left out. This is ongoing.

Learning how autistic women move through the world has been eye-opening and affirming. At last – at LAST – my (apparently) weird personality and traits, and my endless, various struggles are more transparent. Autism is a condition of anxiety and sensitivity, it's about an individual bumping up against social norms and expectations that feel uncomfortable and alien. That hurts – it causes a living dissonance, and makes it difficult to be in the world, and to communicate well with other people.

Like many autistics, I struggle around abstract concepts and social communication. We sometimes miss the subtleties and social conventions that come naturally to neurotypicals. This may be why I have repeatedly ended up in prickly relationship and friendship situations. I would take people at face value, believe all they said or promised, and then become utterly confused and bereft when I misunderstood, or was let down. And I wasn't a skilled communicator of my own needs. Added to that, *I am not like them*, ran through my head all my life – still does sometimes. Ditto: I do not fit / I will never fit / I'm too awkward / Too sensitive / A triangle in a world that loves circles / I annoy everyone / I find people frustrating / They don't understand me / I don't understand them / I'm all out of whack / Life is too hard.

With my diagnosis, the narrative has changed:

I *am* different but there are valid reasons for that / I need to live on my own terms / I need to flow not bend /

There are others like me / Life is hard and beautiful / Self-compassion is crucial / Balance is the goal / What works for neurotypicals does not work for me. And that's A-OK.

My late father used to tell the story of me, as a small child, climbing into his lap and warmly saying, 'Don't we love us?' I have always had a large capacity for love. It's tied in with my empathic nature – something traditionally thought to be missing in autistic people – and it's why I am such an intense friend. I go all in. I love hard. Often, I have been too much, for the love object and for myself. I bombard my new friend or lover; I figure out what they enjoy and offer it up materially – on-point presents; links to articles; themed greeting cards. But intensity is unsustainable, from both sides. And it takes a particularly patient and understanding person to accept, and deal with, my friendship and love. After initial intensity, I often back away, blow a bit hot–cold, begin to assess, but usually my coolness is temporary – I just need some retreat time – and I *will* return if the person can wait. Often, for me, they have not.

People – being around them – causes overwhelm in me. Like many autistics, I don't enjoy group activities, and I don't like talking on the phone, though I love one-on-one, in-person meet-ups, where just we two can natter and set the world to rights. And I like written correspondence, too: texts, emails, cards, letters. But some friends want regular meet-ups, and endless phone conversations, and are disconcerted when I do not; I've lost at least one close friend over this difference in communication styles.

Friendship – and my trickiness around it – has occupied my mind as a central conundrum for some years. I have found it a painful, hard-to-fathom aspect of my life. I've wondered if my high standards have ruined friendships – do I expect way too much of people? Perhaps my strict principles for myself leak over onto others. Maybe I'm too demanding. A nitpicker. Or has my general full on-ness, my blurting of things, and my temporary hermiting confused friends, and driven them away? And have I required understanding of my own up-and-down tendencies, my hot-cold-hot nature, when I didn't understand it all fully myself?

I think some friendships may have been affected by the negative feedback I have experienced since childhood, about outbursts and behaviours associated with impulsivity, and so on. The narrative in my head is one of wrongness because I know I've messed up in the past. When I perceive myself as having said or done the odd/untoward thing (yet again), I withdraw from friends to figure things out, leaving them – potentially – bewildered and irritated. Or, indeed, I may have said/done the wrong things and hurt people unintentionally.

As a sensitive person, I'm also easily wounded. I have moved through friendships over the years and come out the other side scathed and baffled by things said, and done, to me. I've also had a pattern of leaving friendships behind, confined to their time, geography, or situation – school, college, workplaces – with little attempt to extend them onward. Often, the only thing I had in common with the person was the environment where the friendship began. My brain seems to concoct finish lines for friendships – that person doesn't belong in this cordoned-off section of my life, therefore they shall not cross over. It's not that I dislike people – though they often confuse me – it's that I have trotted off to pastures new and things are different here. Or some troubling thing has happened between us that I've interpreted a certain way and I'm brambled in confusion by it. I've realised too late, often, that other people's interpretations of a situation might be different.

For autistics, a shared common interest is often the glue that bonds friendships, and writers/creatives fit that for me. Most of my friends and acquaintances are other writers and artists – we have an instant communion that is valuable and nurturing. Former friendships that were situational didn't have that glueyness, I suppose, the extra something to make them stick.

It is probably no coincidence that my most intimate friends live abroad – the ones that I can spill my heart to in safety. We communicate most usually by email and letter, through social media, and occasional in-person meet-ups. Many of those friends are also older than me. I've always loved old people; from a child I haunted the houses of adult neighbours and relatives, because I enjoyed hearing their stories and learning from them. There was safety around older people for me, I trusted them and found them undemanding in ways that my peers were not.

Giving up alcohol at the age of fifty, along with my subsequent autism diagnosis, has forced an amount of clarity on me. My growth in the four years since removing alcohol from my world has been life-changing; it has precipitated the journey back to the self I abandoned at eighteen, when I first began to Dutch-courage myself into feeling 'on' with people, gregarious, and therefore 'normal'. Without the fug of booze and its attendant dross – impulsivity, precarious situations, rotten hangovers and so on – I see things in general more clearly, including friendships. I better understand my role in failed relationships now; I see why I was a poor friend at times and a poor picker of friends, too. I was so busy masking and pretending in friendships that I didn't explain or represent myself well; I was hiding from others as much as myself. I didn't, or couldn't, set boundaries, or make my needs known, without a lot of agitation. So, I smothered my preferences – for quiet time, for the need to be heard – or demanded them in unhelpful ways, like crying and shouting, or freezing people out.

Because I have the autistic tendency towards naivety and gullibility, and because I'm a helper, I've been quashed by some people in the past. I have been unskilled in protecting myself from bad actors. I often wanted to be amenable, to help others with their pain and issues, rather than acknowledging, or tending to, my own. But my compassion was sometimes taken for granted and, worse, used up by people, so that there was little left for myself.

In one long friendship I was the ever-listening ear, the steady shoulder, the thoughtful giver, and I ended up resentful when that care was never really reciprocated. After time spent with this friend, I would be strung out and exhausted from absorbing their stuff. I hadn't had a chance to share anything of my own, because I was being talked *at* the whole time. When my father died, and that friend stonewalled me, I'd had enough. *Where is the balance,* I asked myself, *the care? Is this person interested in* me *at all?*

I lost my best friend to cancer – my sister Nessa – and two other close friendships have gone by the wayside in recent years, including the one mentioned above. The second of those friend-losses hurt like hell for a time; we were quite alike – both creative loners with anxiety issues – and we bonded empathically and well. But I think I was too much for her, in a variety of ways. Though I confronted that friend when she backed off, she denied she was retreating. Soon she was just a silent speck on the horizon of my life and, it seemed, that was all the answer I was going to get. I've worked hard on accepting her withdrawal, and I think of her fondly, but her absence is felt still.

Anyhow, in ways I've become less tolerant in older age and sobriety – if friends can't take my failings and quirks with my excellence, well, so be it. And even though I may have let people down, and been let down in turn, or I might disagree with a former friend's values, or question their actions, I still love them, if only from afar. My regard for people I once liked and loved rarely dies. I don't give myself easily and I don't require oodles of friends; I'm happiest with a handful of close people. But, because I have few confidants, losing a valued friend leaves a marked gap.

When the two friendships already alluded to ended, I went through a grief phase, really lamenting my lack of super-close friends. But I have my husband, my children (two of them grown men); my siblings, and a few groups I attend. I have online friends to chat with daily, and I also meet other writers in person quite regularly at literary events. And I have a new friend. A sober friend. And she is warm, deep, and perfectly imperfect, just like myself. That is enough sociability for a person who struggles socially.

The combination of Alcohol Out/Autism Affirmation In has brought me home to myself. In the last few years – after a lifetime of befuddlement – I've found I belong right here in this body, and in this mind, uncomfortable and challenging as that can be. Like most people, I'm ever-changing and evolving, still happily learning. Self-care efforts – deep research/taking courses – are teaching me that setting boundaries for myself and with others, and being self-compassionate in the process, is not indulgent or selfish, but completely necessary. All I can do, to be sane and safe, is keep my balance, and try not to skew left or right, but stay to the middle and slow down. Equilibrium is my goal, but it can be an elusive place; when I find that equitable spot, it feels good, but it is also rare.

And, in this new project of being less swing-swongy, I'm more judicious about friendship. I'm dialling back my intensity and stepping slowly with new people; I ease in; I give less freely; I try not to expect much. I want to be treasured for what I bring to relationships (loyalty/care/kindness); I don't want to be moulded into what I am not (ever available/without needs). If certain friends repeatedly upset and tip me over into behaviours or places that I don't value or enjoy, they're not friends I need. If someone retreats and can't say why, well that's OK, too. Perfection doesn't exist, in me or in anyone else.

As I work on reducing control, I'm attempting not to future-predict, and to allow for humps in life and in friendships. Lately I often chant 'what is, what is' when I find myself catastrophising, or trying to foresee outcomes, or understand others' inexplicable behaviours. I learned 'what is' from the glorious Anne Lamott who encourages herself, when she's doom-thinking, not to concentrate on the what-ifs, but on the what-ares. 'What is, what is' reminds me that now is enough and so am I. This kind of compassionate self-talk helps me halt and question that voice, the one that feels shame around being/doing/looking/sounding wrong. The chatterer who delivers negative sentences like, 'You're not good' / 'You won't be able to do this right' / 'You're making mistakes.'

I try hard now to use a considerate tone – encouraging, coaxing – much as I've used with my kids, knowing they respond better to that than haranguing, harsh words. I'm less inclined to babble negatively in my own ear, more able to employ grace and tenderness in my handling of myself. I want to be my own kindest, mother-like, best friend, gently steering myself on. My cart hits inevitable potholes, but I'm slowly acquiring better steadying skills, and I feel more confident by the day that if I take my time, I can catch any falling apples, throw them back into the cart, and travel on in hope.

Jane Cadman was officially diagnosed with autism when she was sixty-nine. She is now seventy-one. Having retired, she is re-imagining and living her whole life from the positive experience of being autistic rather than as an inadequate and confused neurotypical.

Autistic at Seventy

I was nearly seventy when I got my diagnosis for autism, although I had suspected it for several years.

Autism did not exist when I was a child, unless it was extreme male autism. My behaviour would have been considered odd and was subtly corrected. As a child I was paranoically shy. I could not talk to people; I grew up being frighteningly aware that I had to watch my behaviour and what I said. I believe my mother was autistic too. I think she treated all 'strange' behaviour as either naughty (meltdowns or tantrums) or dangerous because it suggested mental illness. She strongly differentiated between behaviour in a social setting and behaviour at home. Strange behaviour outside was not tolerated as it made her feel out of control herself. I think she was teaching me to mask for my own safety. At home she allowed 'eccentricities' but only if they didn't upset her routine. At some level she accepted I was what I was and this gave me a certain confidence in my own identity, even if it was different to others. I remember one rainy day when I was about ten, being fed up with the noise in the house (I had brothers). So I went outside in the rain with my book and built myself a tent from some old canvas in the shed so I could have some peace. I loved the sensory experience of the sound of the rain on the canvas and the dim light. When she eventually found me (I think I was aware of her calling for me in the house, but

I ignored it) she said, 'What a strange child you are.' But it didn't feel like a criticism, more of an acceptance and even admiration for being so self-sufficient. I learnt not to depend on other people's opinions, even my mother's.

I enjoyed learning at school, but not socialising. I never 'understood' the other girls (I went to an all-girls school). I wondered why being around people was so easy for others, but I found it confusing. I had a couple of friends at school and was quite happy with them, but never mixed as the other girls all seemed incomprehensible. I accepted that what went on in my mind was a separate thing to what went on in the social world. To me other people were only relevant as a background to what I was interested in. I learnt social rules as much as I was able and could follow a 'script' of appropriate behaviour. I became very good at masking and assumed that that was what socialising was about. But it always left me with a gap between who I was in myself and other people and a need to get away from them to relax. I accepted a level of loneliness.

I withdrew into books (although I had been reading since I was four and always had to have a book with me throughout my childhood). I could retreat into its world, and both ignore others and be ignored. I went on to do a degree in anthropology. This gave me a perspective on social events and functions. I think I approached my life as if I were an anthropologist studying a strange tribe. My undiagnosed autism, however, prevented me from engaging in society. I was never interested in a career, although I considered becoming a solicitor. But some part of me knew I would not be able to deal with the social aspects of it. The stress would be too much, and I was not interested in doing something for 'social status' reasons. Most of my jobs allowed me to be socially invisible while I filled my life with whatever interested me. Like finds like and throughout my life many of my friends and relationships were with people who were probably neurodivergent and who shared my interests.

About seven years ago I was watching a news item on television. It was about undiagnosed autism in women. They had a woman who had been diagnosed at the age of thirty-four. She described how when she was at work, she followed certain 'social scripts', but she never socialised with her colleagues, like going to the pub, because after work she had to go home and 'reset'. My jaw hit the ground. Here was someone who was describing me exactly. I thought I was the only one who had to do this. I had accepted that I needed to behave like this, but thought I was alone.

I started to research the whole topic (thank goodness for Google!). The more I learnt, the more I was convinced I was autistic. It explained everything, although the work of actually understanding what it means in everyday life is a continuous struggle. It gives a meaningful framework on which to hang my issues without blaming myself for being stupid or wrong. My sensory and processing problems have not gone away, but I am able to develop different strategies to deal with them.

I had lived my social life either with neurodivergent people or behind a mask. It was very easy for me to just pretend. It was automatic. I also realised that although I am good with the written word, I am quite non-verbal. As I got older and came to understand the effect being autistic had on my processing abilities, the lag between my brain and verbalising got slower and I could function with a script, but not if I had to actually connect with what I was thinking and feeling. I think in images, and translating them into words is quite difficult. Over the years the masking had prevented me from negotiating my own emotions and feelings in social settings. This came at a huge cost to my mental health. So even though that masking had allowed me to function relatively well in a neurotypical world, masking as a survival strategy became a problem.

Recognising masking has helped me understand the difference between emotions and feelings. Physiological reactions to external stimuli (emotions, that I sense in my body) are where I become overwhelmed and generally I become stuck in a flight or fight response, which manifests as anxiety or confusion. In a social environment I have no emotional boundaries and do not know whether the emotions are mine or other people's. Masking is how I controlled this maelstrom. I withdrew behind scripts and used my mind to assess appropriate responses. I was never able to go beyond the panic and confusion to become aware of my own feelings separate from what I perceived in others. For instance, if someone asks me whether I like their dress, I do not know what I feel about it or at least not until much later when I have had time to process the visual stimuli; by which time my feelings are irrelevant and therefore to be ignored, leading to ruminating and negative feelings of being 'wrong'. I just know that I have to give an appropriate response at the time and then forget developing feelings about it as they are no longer shareable. Mental health issues come from being disconnected from that process of having an emotional reaction and becoming aware of the feeling and naming it, whether it is anger, grief or even joy. I take a long time to process it so I can never be entirely 'present' in a social interaction. This is exhausting.

Three years ago, at the age of sixty-eight, I became very depressed and suicidal. My husband had died three years before and I could not seem to process it, or rather I seemed to be grieving for all the losses in my life, including being an undiagnosed autistic. I felt as if there was an abyss between myself and others and was overwhelmed by a feeling that I didn't know who I was anymore. I went to my GP, who is very empathetic and understanding. She referred me to the HSE services. I was contacted by the Psychiatry of Later Life Service. I was seen by a psychologist who assessed me for dementia. Thankfully this was not my problem. It was one of the things I was worried about – that I was losing my mind. It is my mind that has seen me through a life that is different from the norm and until then allowed me to work rationally through my difficulties. Being depressed had overwhelmed me emotionally. I did not know why and I could not cope. Self-harm seemed the only way out.

During that session with him, however, which was interesting (I had told him I thought I was autistic), he leaned forward into my personal space and told me I wasn't autistic. I think he meant well, he was trying to be inclusive, make me feel that I wasn't alone. This was well-meaning gaslighting and obviously made me feel more alone, confused and angry. Of course I didn't process all that until at least the day after the session. At the time I just knew that he was wrong. However, he referred me to the HSE Traumatic Bereavement Counselling Service. After a few months' wait, I spent a year with a very good counsellor who accepted my viewpoint and worked from there. It helped a lot.

As part of the counselling process, I decided to get a formal diagnosis. It has given me much greater confidence in my own instincts.

After that event in my life I became concerned about future interactions with mental health and other medical professionals. Although I came through this interaction positively, I am aware that neurotypical people have a serious problem with understanding neurodiversity. Neurodivergent culture is as confusing to them as neurotypical social expectations and understanding are confusing to us.

I was also aware that interwoven with the autism issue was the 'invisible old person' issue. I wonder how many other undiagnosed autistic women of my age and older have added to their problems through their interactions with these uninformed professionals?

Although I did not understand the reasons I felt so different, I think it helped that my mother taught me that social demands were completely separate from my sense of my own individual life journey within the limits of that world. My sense of who I was was not my social identity and the former was mine to discover with or without the 'permission' of social expectation. None of it was easy and many times I felt overwhelmed by that difference. However, I think the sheer cussedness of being (unknowingly at the time) autistic gave me strength and hope. Who I am includes my secret self. I am not a social identity, I do not have to be named or socialised and I continue to evolve.

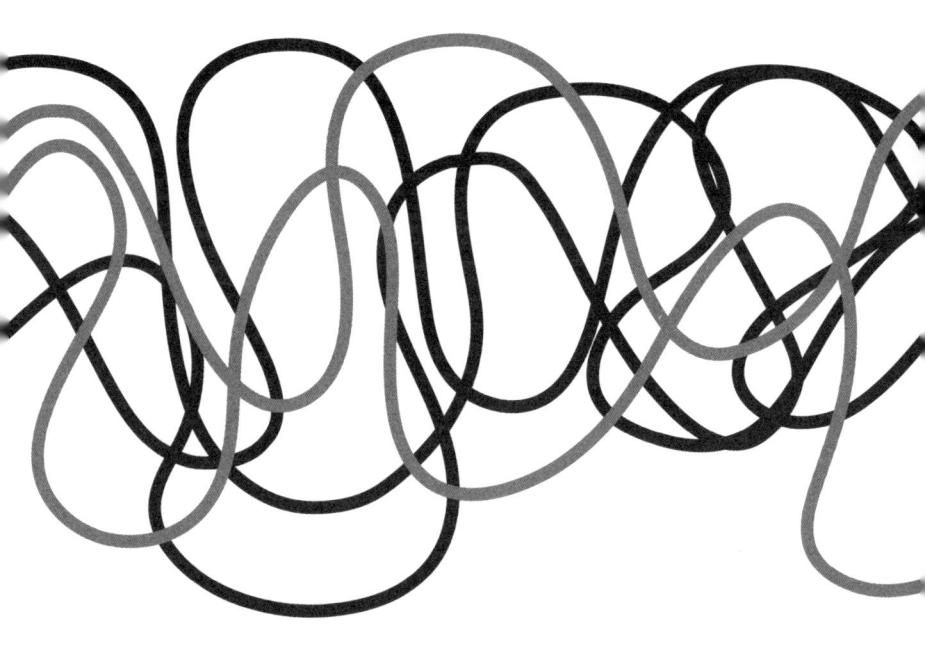

Eric Crowley is an autistic card maker and illustrator, who was diagnosed as a child but didn't find out until he was thirty-three. He lives in Cork City with his family.

Growing

Tell us a bit about yourself.
l have been living in Cork all my life. l am thirty-six and I'm currently working as a production assistant. During my time off I am a graphic designer/illustrator.

When did you learn that you are autistic?
Growing up in Cork city l have always felt 'different'; from my family, friends and other people. During Covid I heard the term 'on the spectrum' on YouTube, and a lot of things fell into place: the schools I was in, my interests, my fear of groups and my preferring to be alone.

My heart sank when I asked both my mom and dad, separately, if I had autistic tendencies. I was diagnosed as autistic at the age of four. Both Mom and Dad had very different things to say about it. My mom couldn't understand it as much, and was optimistic I would grow out of it if my family accepted me for me, but I always knew I was 'different'.

This was in 1989 and the knowledge of autism was unspoken of back then. I think my dad was a bit relieved as he thought that maybe he could find an answer to help me. I was fussy with food. My concentration was poor and I would not eat anything unless I was watching TV, and had to be spoon-fed for a while. My dad picked up on this when I was very young, and Mom thought I was a bit slow or late to learn new things, and eventually I would grow out of it.

There was one movie called *Rain Man*, Dustin Hoffman's character had autism as well. I think my parents were afraid I would end up like that character.

I understand it was a different time and my parents handled it the best they could. They were scared I might not turn out the way they imagined and have a future: getting a job, meeting new people and enjoying life. Instead I would have been searching for help from doctors and psychologists, looking for as much as I could. I was looking for support, and understanding of myself.

I wish they told me a bit sooner. I would have handled it better instead of comparing myself to others and 'not fitting in'. Both my parents were afraid of how I would react until I asked them. But they are happy how I turned out.

What do you think about how the media portrays autistic people?
I have watched shows like *Love on the Spectrum* and it broke me. I related to some of the characters, but words like 'being normal', or the one I hate is 'one of a kind'. I think people still see us as a hindrance or something to look after.

I haven't seen many autistic people in animation yet and I would like to see it but am very worried about which direction it would take.

What was your experience of school?
I was sent to a 'special school' called Scoil Triest in Cork City. During my time at Scoil Triest I was evaluated for my speech and language skills. I was quiet growing up, and went to a lot of speech therapy from the age of four.

My understanding of language and vocabulary had improved over time, and I was recommended to attend a class for children with a language disorder, and both my parents agreed to this.

Around the age of seven I went to study at a mainstream school as I had improved my social skills and was adjusting to bigger classrooms of people. I had one-to-one classes for extra learning in maths and in English, as the goal was to move me to a school closer to home.

Secondary school did not change much. I wanted to get a job early, as hanging around after school was boring. I wanted to keep myself busy. I was meant to be taken out of mainstream school a second time, but I adjusted, and later learnt I was masking. I did all the things other kids did, like wearing soccer jerseys. I pretended to like soccer, and later on I went to nightclubs and other social gatherings like everyone else.

You say you pretended to like soccer, but what interests did you really have?
I didn't play sport, as I thought it was very aggressive and it was too serious, and to this day I still don't.

I had a hyper-fixation on video games. People say they have a drive or passion. It's not that at all; I'm doing it to keep me happy, and to not fall into a ball of depression.

Learning about different animation styles led me to discover anime and manga. I kept quiet about this and only talked about it with very close family and friends. This was in 2007 and I remember anime and manga weren't as well received as most popular cartoons back then, whereas today anime and manga are more popular than ever, and have a genre for everyone, e.g. romance, horror and sci-fi to name a few.

Wired Our Own Way

What did you do after secondary school?
After secondary school I studied animation, and a few years later I studied graphic design. In my college years I finally had a place I could call home in animation, as drawing was my passion. The students and I had a lot in common, but I was torn trying to please everyone. I enjoyed college, made new friends, and joined a few societies. I managed college independently. But sometimes the college and part-time job balance was hell.

What has your love of anime, drawing and manga done for you?
I have met a lot of artists around Ireland by going to anime conventions. These conventions introduced me to so many new experiences and new things, and I have more online friends now, which is great.

My exercise routine came from watching anime. I watched shows and saw characters working out in gyms and practising more peaceful exercises like yoga and tai chi. Yoga was a great release for me, the silence in the room and slow movements are very soothing.

Are there things you find hard about socialising?
Being in big groups of people is very difficult for me and this is where l can be quiet the most, as l don't know when my cue is to add to a discussion, and when l do speak I tend to trail off.

People say I am too honest for my own good. I was taught by my parents not to lie, and so I freeze in conflict so I don't create trouble for myself. I am afraid to speak my mind, and as a result I sit alone to protect myself.

I want to be more approachable, as I have been told I am very kind, thoughtful and caring. Maybe it's because

I sit on my own and draw or read, and people think I'm arrogant or snobbish. But I can't help who I am and why should I have to justify that? I had to stand up for myself after being ghosted and feel absolutely miserable because of it, for just being me.

My social circle is much smaller now than it was in my teenage years but I have yet to find my 'tribe', but I have met more friends online through my artwork.

How is life now?
I have come a long way. I have travelled around the country on my own. I have made work to sell. I have worked on a video game called *No Straight Roads* but I don't play video games as much these days. I spend my time improving my art skills and these have opened my social circle even more. I work full time and am a graphic designer and illustrator in my spare time.

I have taken up new classes in yoga and tai chi, and I go to the gym. I talk to a therapist every other week.

Relationships are very few. I haven't dated anyone in five years and I'm not bothered. If it happens, that's great, but it's not a main priority.

I am terrified for the future, of getting a place for myself. I am now pushing myself in work, and in my art outside of work. Having a place of my own where I can work from home is my goal. I am the eldest in my family and both my younger siblings are doing better than me and have moved out of my parents' house.

Although now I am very comfortable talking about being on the spectrum I am still learning, and have felt as if being autistic is used against me. There are days and they are awful, like work issues.

Is there anything you would change if you went back in time?
If I went back in time, maybe to my twenties, I would have requested my files from Scoil Triest then. I am very happy that I have them now. The school was very pleasant and understanding to work with. I'm glad. I'm incredibly lucky to have the information as getting diagnosed nowadays is a nightmare.

Have you any advice for other people with similar experiences to you?
I can't give any advice as my experiences will be different to others, but try what works for you. Talking about it is the very first thing that will help in the long run.

I went for therapy in 2018 and it did wonders for me: learning about myself and trying all sorts of helpful things and discussing difficult topics. I learnt different techniques to help me feel safe: meditation, breathing exercises and discovering the inner child. It helps me to take small steps into achieving what I want in life and to find people who I can relate to.

Fear of the unknown had plagued my mind in the past, and I overcame this in little ways and have made life-changing decisions on my own and I am very proud of that. I am hoping to meet others like me as it would help me and hopefully others who have gone through a similar experience.

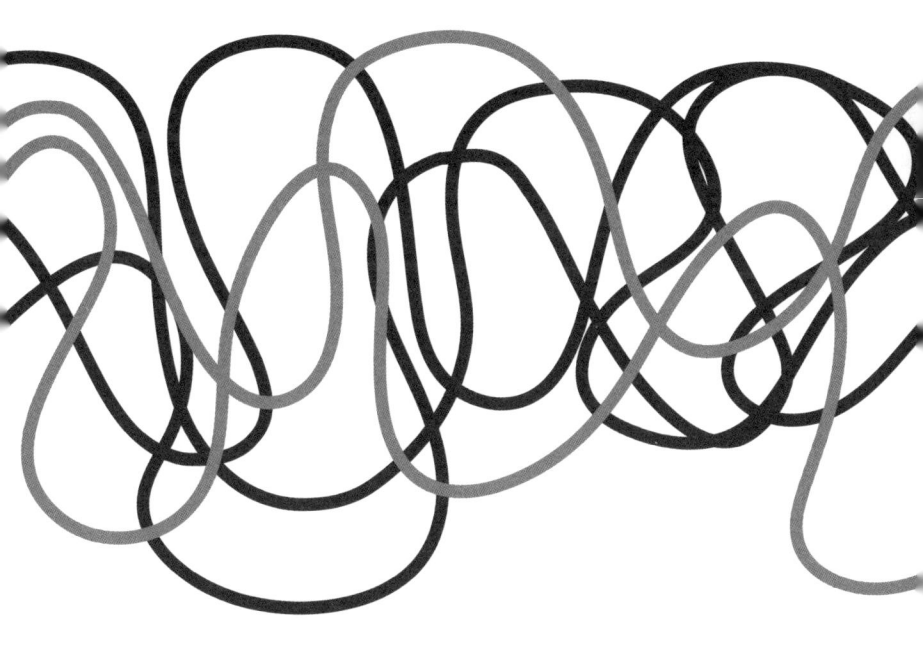

James McClean is a professional footballer who played 103 games for the Republic of Ireland, as well as featuring for Sunderland, West Brom, Wigan Athletic, Stoke City, Wrexham and Derry City. James was diagnosed with autism at thirty-three and has a daughter, Willow-Ivy, who is also autistic.

Discovering Autism

Autism was something that I never knew too much about, even though it had been with me forever. I was diagnosed as autistic in 2023, having had our daughter Willow-Ivy diagnosed previously.

When I decided to go through the diagnosis process, it was because there were so many similarities between Willow and me. I had thought about it for a long time, particularly watching Willow grow up, seeing her little ways, her little differences to her older siblings and recognising that her family was her 'safe space'.

Willow-Ivy is an incredible little girl.

Like many parents of autistic children, we feared the worst when Willow was diagnosed. Not that she wouldn't be accepted, but more so that all the challenges she would face as she grew up would be difficult for her. Automatically, your mind goes to: 'Will she have friends?'; 'How will she get on in school?'; 'How will she be when she's older?'; 'Who will look after her if she needs someone?'

Her relationship with her siblings is something that we are most proud of, not just because of how understanding and loving Allie-Mae, Junior and Mia are, but because of how comfortable and safe Willow feels with them. It is with them where she can be anything and still be loved. She can be herself, she can play, she can laugh, she can throw tantrums with them, and they don't treat her any differently.

When she needs her quiet time, they give her it. When she wants to have fun and a laugh with them, they do that too.

That's something myself and my wife Erin are very proud of.

I was never aware of autism, only knowing a handful of people who may have had someone autistic in their family. But in terms of the sensory and social challenges it presented, I was not well-versed. I know a number of people who have autistic children, and their interests are concentrated on one or two things, whether it's music, video games, technology, and so on. And in my own case it is, and always has been, football. I was kicking a ball for as long as I can remember.

Being a footballer was all I ever wanted to do. I had no interest in school, and instead was fixated on playing football in any setting. Being from a close-knit community like Creggan, you grow up learning to be streetwise, and a lot of that came from being out on the streets with a ball.

I signed for my hometown club, Derry City, in 2008 and after a couple of successful seasons I moved to Sunderland, who were in the Premier League at the time. It was my first time living away on my own. It was my first time being away from my family and in a city where I knew nothing and nobody. Every weekend I would try get a late flight home after a match just to get back for a day. Failing that, my friends would come over and spend the weekend with me.

It was a challenge because I had never had to cook, or clean, or discover a new place before like that. But over time and alongside Erin, we adapted with the different moves I made and found somewhere we and the kids call 'home'. That allowed me to keep a focus on my career.

When I got to my twenties I began to add that bit extra to my approach to football. I became obsessed with training and improving. I looked at the tiny details of what I was doing, and how I could get better and how I could continue to stay at the top of my game. I train several times a day between the pitch and the gym. Sometimes, when I'm bored, I'll get my running shoes on and get out and train. Anytime we have moved house in England, the most important part of it has always been the gym.

I go there and get my head down for an hour. It's just me against me there. Every bit of struggle or pain that I feel during a session, I just keep going. Because tough work makes tough people.

Routine is another thing. Like so many autistic people, routine is something that is very important in my life. That's where being a footballer helps. Our weeks are never too different, we train and we play a match home or away, that's the way it is. You then have your time built around that. Most of mine is at home with my family.

Socially, I have my family, my close friends and my teammates and that is enough. Anyone that knows me on a personal level knows that I am quiet, a bit introverted and enjoy my own company. I like nothing more than sitting with a can of Red Bull and watching any kind of football or boxing that may be on. It has become part of my routine, and again, it is something that made me think about the traits that Willow and I share. I do not do nights out. I never thought about it, but the sensory aspect of a night out may have contributed to that. The noise, the lights, the people shouting over each other, banging into each other. Give me a night in front of the TV anytime.

My social battery is not the highest – truthfully, I sometimes avoid situations that I may find challenging in a social capacity. Things like large gatherings, weddings, parties, they have never been my scene. My friends will tell you the same. With them, I am fine. We slag each other but look out for each other, and every day you find something else to laugh about. But outside of that, it's fair to say not many people engage with me on a day-to-day basis.

When I had the chance to align with AsIAm (Ireland's national autism charity) earlier this year, I wanted to make sure that we as a family put ourselves alongside it. We will move back to Ireland in the next few years, and it is organisations like AsIAm, ones that are doing tireless work to support people and families with autism, that will become a part of our life when we do.

But overall, I am proud to be autistic. It is something that makes me, me. It is something that further connects me and Willow, and will let her know that no matter what challenges she ever faces, her daddy can help her, along with her mammy, brother and sisters. I think that a lot of my career can be attributed in some way to my traits – I am obsessed with football. Training and getting fitter, faster and stronger is something that has been in me for years.

I never want Willow to be afraid of chasing her dreams. I would hate for autistic people to think that chasing their dreams is something they cannot do. That is another reason why I am so proud to be autistic and hopeful that somebody will be inspired by what I have done in my career. Autism is a part of you, but it should not define what you can and cannot achieve – whether it is playing for your country, or becoming a parent, or getting the best marks in exams (I was never good at that!), or becoming a doctor, or anything else.

It is something that makes you special, the best kind of special. And I have a daughter that is the best kind of special and inspires me every single day.

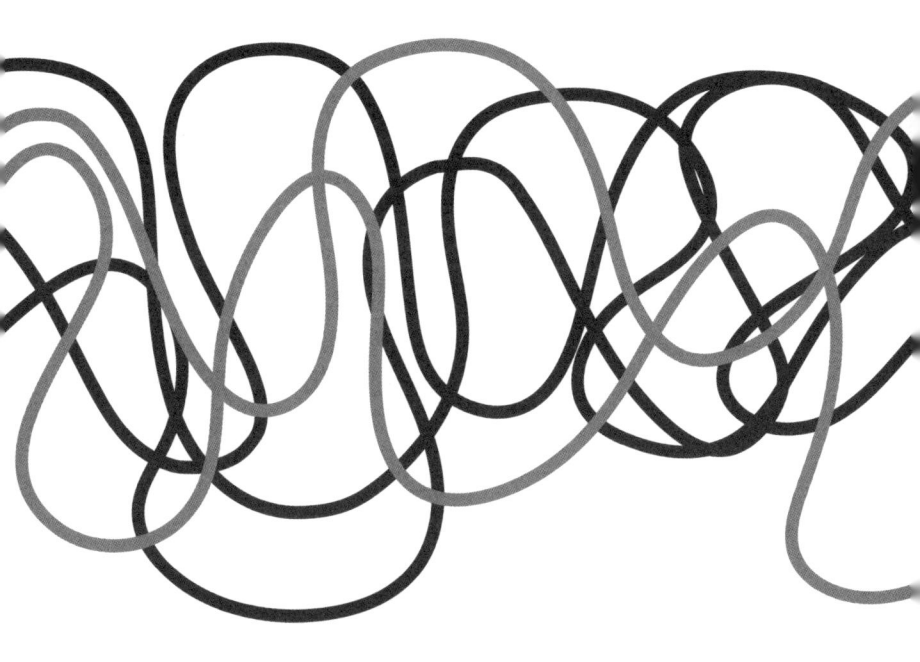

Róisín Riley is eighteen and is studying for a BA in applied psychology at University College Cork. Róisín loves to read and believes in the importance of creating a more autism-affirming world after receiving her recent autism diagnosis.

Thirteen

I was thirteen when my mum died. My four older siblings and I were brought into a family room in the intensive care unit of Galway Hospital, where my mum was being treated. I remember everybody crying after a lady spoke, who I could not determine to be a nurse, social worker or some other comforting authoritative figure. I remember walking down a corridor so modernly designed that it should not have been as dark as it was. I remember being confused about why my family were moving so slowly when we were going in to see our mum in intensive care. Why would they not walk faster? She was so sick, where was the urgency to see her while she was still alive? It was almost frustrating. I did not understand.

When I close my eyes today, I'm still walking into that dim, compartmented room where my mum was. The flames of tealights mocked me, the machines that beeped so eagerly just yesterday stood quiet. My mum was there, but she was dead.

I did not understand, walking in there, that she would be dead. I thought she was still alive.

Nobody had explicitly told me the word 'dead' so I did not fathom that death was a possibility. The person you need most in the world is dying: how did I not realise that was what had happened? I felt like an idiot: all my siblings had known, they had understood, yet I had walked into that room expecting to say goodbye to my mum. I knew to expect something bad, but I hadn't heard the word 'dead', so did not assume the death had already occurred. I had not even begun to consider it as a possibility. Yet she was already dead.

You may be wondering, what does this have to do with being autistic? I feel that now I'm aware that I am, and always have been, an autistic girl, every facet of each of my life experiences links back to me being autistic.

I was not diagnosed as autistic until I had just turned eighteen, and it was then that I was able to look back on the day I lost my mum through a fresh lens. I feel so deeply for that thirteen-year-old girl. She was not silly for not realising her mum had died; she just had a very literal way of thinking. She was not reacting 'wrong' when she couldn't comprehend that her mum had died until years later; her brain just had a different way of processing information.

All these things could be dismissed as a typical reaction to such a bereavement for a thirteen-year-old. But I know now that there is a difference. Now that I am aware of being autistic, it seems that almost every occurrence in my life is explained. It is as if I was in a dark room, stumbling and tripping over clutter that I couldn't see. But now the light is on. The room is no tidier, it is actually still quite a mess. But the light is on, so I can see the clutter; I can begin to tidy it all up now.

My entire life, I have never known what it is that I feel or think. When the word 'alexithymia' and its meaning, 'significant challenges in recognising, expressing and describing emotions', was first introduced to me, a huge lamp in that dark room was switched on.

I have always had great difficulty in identifying and understanding my own emotions. I went on to learn that I was never grieving 'wrong' in not knowing how to even begin to assimilate my emotions, I simply had alexithymia. My incredibly thoughtful and caring brother has asked me during times where my mental health has been at its lowest, 'What would you say if "I don't know" wasn't an option?' In his attempts to encourage me to share my feelings he received nothing other than an 'I don't know' and tears of frustration in response. It may have seemed that I was being defiant – and I have often been described as not wanting to bother other people by telling them what I'm feeling – but the reason behind my refusal to divulge my emotions has always been exactly what I've told people: I don't know what they are. How would you describe how you are feeling to somebody when you yourself don't even know what it is that you're feeling? How would you share your thoughts if you had no idea what those thoughts were?

It is frustrating to sit in therapy being asked what it is that I'm feeling, what I've been doing, what I've been thinking, what triggers these things, and only being able to say 'I don't know.' I'm not being uncooperative, I'm not holding back on sharing. I just genuinely and truly do not know, and I wish I did.

For my entire life, I've had alexithymia but did not know what it was. 'No words for emotions' is the descriptor that was given to me by the psychiatrist who first introduced the term to me. He coincidentally went on to diagnose me as autistic, simultaneously giving me the identity that I never knew I needed and saving my life. Without meeting me, after only hearing about my encounter with another doctor on his team, he had suggested that maybe I should be assessed for autism.

For just one person to recognise who I was, to suggest that I was the autistic person that I didn't even know I was, changed everything. The uncertainty of who I am had been lifted and while I didn't instantly know all the answers and wasn't magically mentally well and void of all sensory and social difficulties, it made sense. And that is all I needed. I needed to have that light switched on. To understand why I was the way I was, the way I still am. To understand that I don't need to be changed: I need to be *recognised*.

I could continue describing how discovering I'm autistic has bestowed me with resolution and wisdom, but it also prompted many questions, frustrations and angers. Why did it take seventeen years – my entire life – for somebody to question that maybe I was autistic? Somebody I had never even met! Where were the people in my life who were meant to look after me when I was growing up as an autistic girl who displayed many autistic traits? Why did they not see me?

But I know these people are not at fault. I didn't even know that I was autistic, so how were they supposed to? I was not the stereotypical autistic child, so it was never questioned as a possibility. The generalisations of society to view autism through such a narrow lens are harmful to anybody who does not fall under the stereotypes created, and that is a lot of people. Diagnostic criteria that are biased and unjust allowed me, and allow many others, to struggle through their entire life undiagnosed and unsupported. How would my autism have been identified if the way I behaved wasn't regarded to be what society perceives as 'autistic'?

My intense fascination with and constant absorption in books was dismissed as a hobby. My difficulties in forming and maintaining friendships were attributed to shyness. My excellence in school dictated me to be a 'gifted' child. My withdrawal after a day of subconsciously masking all aspects of my autism was reduced to me being 'a quiet child'. I could go on. It hurts to think of every day of my life where I went undiagnosed, unrecognised and misunderstood, but I look back now with forgiveness for the confused girl who fought to be the only thing society would accept her to be: 'normal'. I wish I could tell her that she had been normal all along.

I wish I could go back to thirteen-year-old Róisín who walked into the intensive care unit expecting to see her mum alive, when in reality she was dead. I wish I could go back to that girl who did not understand the grave situation because her brain worked differently to everybody else's. I would tell her that she's autistic because she deserves to know that, and that there is nothing bad about that. I would tell her to stay. I would tell her that she will be OK. I would tell her that her voice is needed in this world, and that one day she will recognise that.

I am only eighteen now. I was only diagnosed as autistic a mere few months ago. But I have learnt so much already. I now know that my voice is needed in this world. Thirteen-year-old me lives within me, and I within her, so each day I speak to her in the way that she should always have been spoken to. I tell her that there is nothing wrong with her. Her presence is needed on this planet. Her fighting so heartbreakingly each day just to stay alive is more important than she will ever know.

So I say the same to each autistic person reading this: your voice is needed. Your experiences and feelings are valid and should never be dismissed. I recognise you and I understand you, and the things I don't understand, I accept.

Wired Our Own Way

You are important and I'm sorry if you have ever felt that you aren't. To every person who sees just a small part of themselves in the confused thirteen-year-old girl in that hospital, who can't seem to keep up with everybody else: there is nothing wrong with you. Please, always remember that you are different, not less.

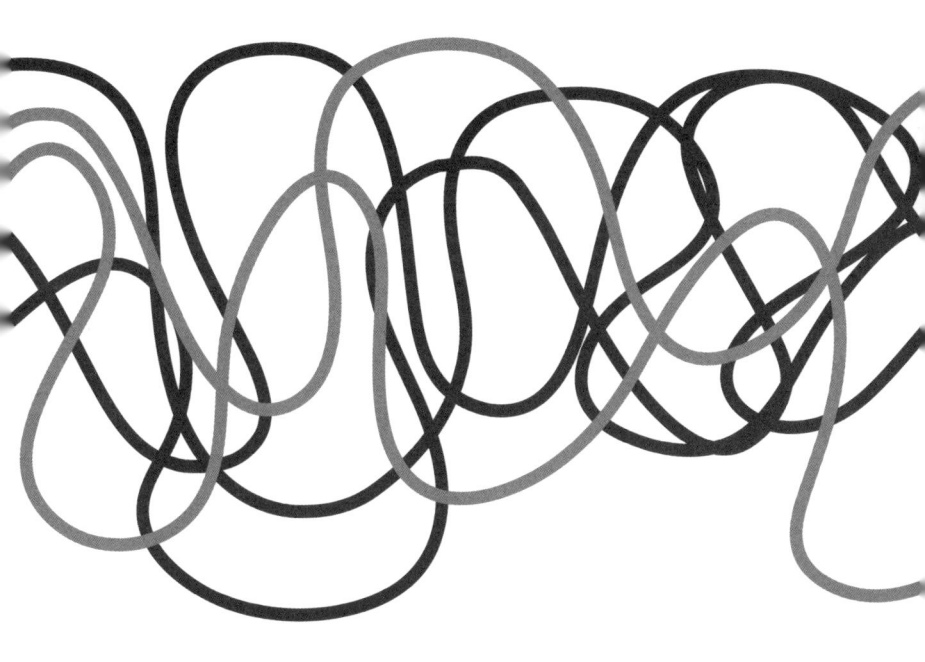

Fiacre Ryan is a young non-speaking autistic writer, poet and disability advocate. He scripted his own award-winning documentary for RTÉ, *Speechless*, and his book of the same name was published by Merrion Press. He lives in Castlebar with his family.

Poetic Justice

P	Pee-ed
O	Off
E	Every
T	Time
I	I
C	Can't
J	Join
U	Uttering
S	Silent
T	Thoughts
I	Intelligent
C	Contributions
E	Easily.

This poet does not speak,
He writes his own rhyme and rhythm,
Beating out ideas to everyone who listens,
And those who don't.
Justice for non-speakers,
Forged in the iron flames of ignorance,
Branded for life,
Dumb.
Burning men's perceptions,
His searing wisdom scorches the unjust.
This poet seeks only that justice,
To be re-branded, unchained,
Free.

Key Words

Definition: Key
- a small piece of shaped metal with incisions which is inserted to open a lock
- buttons on a panel for operating a computer, typewriter or telephone
- of crucial importance

All of these definitions are the sum of my life as an autistic person who uses AAC to communicate. AAC is Augmentative and Alternative Communication, and encompasses all the ways that someone communicates, excluding the spoken word.

The Diagnosis
I was born destined to be silent, with a range of sensory issues and a brain that was somehow wired differently to everyone else I knew. I was diagnosed with autism at around three years of age, and with a mild to moderate learning disability. After early intervention, speech and occupational therapy (mostly sourced by my parents), I graduated to the label of non-verbal to add to my collection. Today I prefer to use the term non-speaking, which I feel describes me more accurately. Some people assume that I am not capable of learning, but my mind is intact in a body that doesn't always co-operate.

Early Life

> See the world through my eyes as I navigate through yours.★

My early years were a rollercoaster ride through the neurotypical world where I searched for the keys to my existence. Keys played an important part in my life as doors, windows and gates had to be locked so that I would not escape from our estate. Keys were elusive hidden objects, secreted away to various hiding places, away from my curious fingers. A key can mean the difference between freedom and imprisonment, or even life and death. For me, a key always meant freedom, a way into another world where my turbulent thoughts and brainstorms could wander and roam, somehow finding their own peace.

Living and Learning

> I glean knowledge by observing my world: looking, imagining, seeing pictures and understanding life.★

Now I had to learn ways to navigate this world that I lived in and survive it. I developed my own ways to communicate, bringing people by the hand to show them what I wanted, pointing, flapping my hands, nodding my head, sometimes screaming on the floor and banging my head in frustration, running away and hiding from unpleasant situations and unpleasant people. Hand-flicking and finger-waving are not generally regarded as indicators of intelligence; stims are something to be eliminated, especially if visitors, inspectors, psychologists or other experts are about. My mam says I brought pictures of Croagh Patrick when I wanted to go climbing or hiking. To communicate that I wanted to go swimming, I would pull out the swim bag and put on my favourite video of myself splashing in water. I used PECS, the Picture Exchange Communication System, visual schedules and later various apps, but all felt limiting, and I yearned once again for that elusive key to free my own meaningful language.

Finding the Key

> My life is totally transformed since I learnt to communicate.*

When I was first introduced to spelling on an alphabet letterboard, I was a downy bird trying to fly, weak, scared, worried, daunted, yet marvelling that I finally knew these ABC letters could set me soaring skywards on worded wings.

Communication takes many forms, from gestures to writing, Post-its, cards, dictating, transcribing, scribing, spelling, pictures, signing, pointing to letters on a letterboard, typing, reading apps and voice-generating apps. The letterboard is my key to communication, for I am one who communicates differently. Even today I am still amazed that everyone can see my words and my sentences as I spell, but it has taken many hours of practice, patience and support to become fluent and achieve open communication. There were many evenings when I laboured at my homework on my letterboard with my sisters at the kitchen table, and I longed for my previous carefree life!

I have to be precise and accurate on the letterboard and iPad and concentrate fully, regulating my body and my mind, for example with compression exercises, so that I can type out meaningful conversations and discussions.

Having a different method of communication brings its own set of problems. A diagnosis of intellectual disability with a lack of communication skills meant that I was underestimated for much of my early years. Some people were reluctant to see past my autistic behaviours and accept that I was intelligent enough to spell words and formulate sentences, even though I had been absorbing language and learning all my life. Some people felt threatened by my ability to express my thoughts and opinions as it didn't suit their own narrative for autism. When I started spelling back the conversations I was listening to, however, people soon stopped talking in front of me as if I wasn't there!

Communication is the key to the doors of inclusion and acceptance, and it has freed the turbulent thoughts in my head. As I lay my thoughts out on a page or a screen, with my chosen voice output, I am finally being respected and understood. I chose my voice from a list of accents, with *Conor's Irish voice* being my best option. I have unlocked my inner voice. Beautiful happenings occur when I escape from the prison of my silence.

With letterboard spelling and typing I am expressing myself daily, and I can show the world my deepest thoughts and feelings. I can join discussions, give my opinions, share my ideas. I can make my own decisions, and convey them to others. I may not always be in control of my body, but I have regained control of my life.

I will tell anyone who will listen, and those who won't, that I am intelligent and that my fellow non-speaking autistics and I understand far more than anyone thinks. I know that our day will come to take our rightful place in society. We yearn for understanding and acceptance in your neurotypical world, our shared world. Sadly it may be too late for some, but we will continue to advocate for others, one letter at a time.

Access to AAC
If non-speaking autistic people are not given access and training in AAC, and provided with a language-based alternative to spoken language adapted to our abilities and skills, we will face significant challenges across many areas in life. We will have difficulties in accessing education, employment, transport, public services, health services, recreational facilities, social opportunities and with living in our own communities. Also, our needs and priorities may change over time, and any supports will need to reflect this, in any plans for our future. A future that we sadly might not have any say in, where our voices are not being heard.

New Autism Research
I am very excited about new research into autism, as the focus is now moving on to studies investigating the abilities of non-speaking, unreliably-speaking and minimally-speaking autistic children and adults in many countries.

I was privileged to take part in the Cambridge University research study *Hidden Cognitive Abilities in Non-Speaking Autism* (woolgarlab.org), using the latest brain-imaging technology to investigate language-processing abilities in non-speaking autistics, as this was an opportunity for me to prove my linguistic abilities.

New assessment methods which do not require a spoken response, such as eye-tracking technology and brain-imaging, have been trialled with AAC users. It is estimated that, worldwide, at least a third of the autistic population is non-speaking, yet very limited research has been carried out up to now on this population, with most of the research focused on the speaking population. The results and recommendations from the verbal cohort research have influenced the education and interventions for a very different population of non-speakers like me.

Research into eye tracking of letterboard users has been published recently, and studies also indicate that non-speaking autistic people's capacity for language and literacy may have been significantly underestimated.

This theory has been explored in the film *The Reason I Jump*, based on the writings of Naoki Higashida, and in the movie *Spellers*, inspired by the book *Underestimated* by Jamie and J. B. Handley.

From my own personal experience, I would suggest that myself and my fellow non-speaking autistics may have been underestimated cognitively, underestimated in language processing, and underestimated in acquiring literacy. Perhaps it is time now to see beyond our autism and presume competence and explore our hidden abilities.

My Key Words

The keys I searched for as a young boy to escape from the turmoil of my days, the keys that led me to a communication method that changed my life, the keys that will help me to type my future, my 'key words' have indeed proved to be of crucial importance to me as I navigate my way through the world. My autism no longer defines me, rather now I can define my own life.

My name is Fiacre, and I am an AAC user.

★ Fiacre Ryan, *Speechless: Reflections from My Voiceless World* (Merrion Press, 2022)

Justin Bakker is an eternal hobbyist. He works in IT and fills his evenings and weekends with a succession of passionate creative interests ranging from musical composition and arrangement, to woodworking, to painting and writing. Originally from the Netherlands, he has been living in Dublin for nearly twenty years.

How Not to Write a Musical Composition

Step 1: Master the trumpet
You're ten years old and you've decided to master the trumpet. You're pretty sure your grandfather played it, but this might have been a misunderstanding. However, your autistic hyperfocus superpower won't let that stop you. You start lessons, and practise daily. First twenty minutes, then an hour. Your parents eventually need to come to an arrangement with the neighbours about when you can practise and for how long, so everyone can get some sleep as well. You remain just as determined as ever.

When you get good enough, you learn that there's such a thing as competitions for musical instruments, and of course you have to enter. Joining the local concert band is next and you become the youngest first chair in the band. The library has a great selection of music books and you try to memorise famous jazz solos, determined to play them flawlessly. This isn't just about learning; it's about immersing yourself in the music, everything else will disappear.

Step 2: Childhood composition
You've been playing the trumpet for two years now, you can hear a grand composition in your head. It's just a matter of getting it on paper. Armed with your 1980s Apple Macintosh Plus and a basic music notation

application, you dive in with high hopes. You're in the zone and spend hours in the library reading sheet music and transcribing everything note for note into the music notation application, hoping this method somehow will teach you how to compose. The melodies come easy enough, you can play them on your trumpet, but you just don't get the theory. No matter how many songs you copy into the application, the breakthrough never comes. Still, you give it your all, even if your masterpiece doesn't make it past eight bars.

Step 3: Scrap the trumpet, guitar is the next thing
The trumpet was great, but now that you are a teenager it's all about the guitar. Sure, you only picked this up to impress a girl, but soon the instrument resonates with you on a much deeper level. You're all in, you find yourself as you lose yourself, working through library books and practising for hours. Blisters on your fingers? They are just battle scars, they will scab over, you'll wear them with pride. Just being able to play a few chords isn't enough, you study bar chords and finger-picking styles. The guitar consumes you fully, you feel a deep engagement. If you're not playing, you're thinking about playing, it's the first thing you do when you get home. Reading guitar tablature has become second nature, when you get stuck you take a few lessons to get you to the next stage, but you keep going until you have truly conquered this instrument.

Step 4: Compose a song
Playing someone else's music is getting boring, you want to work out how to write your own music. You notice that most music uses some variations of the same chords,

so that's a great start. You quickly put a song together and invite a few friends over to record it. The second song doesn't work as well, neither does the third, you keep hitting the limit of your songwriting skills.

The problem is your limited understanding of music theory, the only solution you see is to enrol in a year-long university course. You imagine the course will unlock your potential, but instead you're struggling. Music theory is a lot harder than you imagined. You get through the exam but it drains you. Your excitement for writing songs has long since passed, and with it your passion for the guitar.

Step 5: Become a dancer
Why waste time studying music when you can dance? You discover salsa when you are looking for a salsa band to join and stay to learn the basics of the dance. Never one for half measures, soon you're dancing six nights per week, it's all you can think of. You go to every salsa class you can find, dancing is the only thing that matters right now. When there are no classes you practise at home, studying videos, listening to salsa music. You become known as a good technical dancer who not only masters dancing 'on one', but also the far more technical 'on two'. Who knew there were salsa congresses as well? You dance till your feet are aching and then you keep going. You struggle to walk the next day. You love being in the zone, it's intensely satisfying, it's like nothing else exists and all you are is movement and music.

Step 6: Piano is the new frontier
As expected, your interest in dancing fades, but you've already moved on to a new passion: learning to play the

piano. You buy the instrument, order a book and get on with it. Your fingers start hurting again, as you stretch them in unfamiliar ways. You will make them get used to this, it worked with the guitar, it will work with the piano. You keep practising and bit by bit you get the hang of it. Reading two staves is a bit tricky; your years of trumpet come in handy but you can't read the bass clef fluently. You start to translate guitar chords to piano chords and experiment with chord styles. There's that submersion again, that warm wonderful feeling where everything makes sense. Time is meaningless, sometimes you find yourself at 2 a.m. and you're still playing, where has the time gone?

Step 7: Start painting

OK, maybe piano isn't it after all. After a while, learning the piano started to feel like a chore, and staying motivated became harder. It's difficult to keep up. Why do you feel such an intense interest and then suddenly it's gone? What you need is something that truly captivates you. And after a few months you discover this in painting. You plunge in, squeezing an easel into the cosy sunroom off the kitchen, overfilling the shelves with paintbrushes and oils. When you work on a portrait of your wife you keep telling yourself you'll just spend five more minutes tidying things up. By the time you get up your legs feel stiff and you realise it's 4 a.m. It's relaxing to de-screen and switch off. Research becomes crucial, what palette did Van Gogh prefer? Are there tutorials online on achieving more lifelike skin tones? You set yourself an ambitious goal to create enough artwork to join an exhibition at St Stephen's Green.

Being in the zone is wonderful, and you'll miss it when it's gone. Interests are intense, all-consuming, but you notice they rarely last. This one will fade as well, so you try to enjoy it.

Step 8: Run a marathon or four
Goals keep you motivated, but after a few disappointing paintings you feel your enthusiasm waning. You really love painting, but you no longer feel the passion. You try another painting, but even as you prime the canvas, you struggle. It's no use. The intensity of the interest is gone. You mourn it, for weeks you are restless, looking for something to do, something to sink your teeth into.

You're in your forties now and the need to stay healthy presents you with a new ambition. You've run a bit here and there and you were decent enough at it. You decide to give it a go. But why run a 5k if you can do the marathon? Without too much thought you sign up for the Dublin marathon, and running quickly becomes your new passion. You research training plans, equipment (you don't need a lot, that's good) and race tactics. This really suits you and you start to build some serious endurance. Running quickly goes from the odd run to running five times per week.

This is what you are meant to be doing. Before long, you're talking about fuelling, carb loading and pace like a pro. One marathon turns into four, and you find yourself in the zone once more.

Step 9: Write a composition
Once the marathon is over each year, your running falls off a cliff until the following spring and you're restless, waiting to find something new to sink your teeth in. Music has always been there, lingering in the background. You need to go back to your first goal, you're going to compose that piece

of music. When you were a child you lacked the skills and endurance, but here you are now. Joining the local concert band has brought back the idea of writing a composition. And being who you are, there's no doubt you're going to go for it. You learn everything there is to know about it, from theory of composing to just experiencing again and again your favourite compositions. You take time off work to attend a composition workshop at the National Concert Hall. Guitar and piano taught you about chords, while the trumpet trained your ear for melody. Dancing improved your sense of rhythm, and running marathons, well, that built your stamina.

The beauty of being in the zone
Each passion burns brightly, and then one day, the spark is gone. You've learnt to live with it, to embrace it. Your obsessions never last, but this is who you are. If there's one thing autism has taught you, it's that you have the ability to chase a passion with unwavering enthusiasm and commitment.

Interests may come and go, the beauty lies in the intensity of the moments when you are fully absorbed, when all that matters is music, dancing or painting. It always seems to slip away, and you're dreading the moment when it's gone, but when you're in it, it's yours.

As you rehearse your composition with the local concert band, you're not worried about how long this will last. For now, you're in the zone again, and for now, that's more than enough.

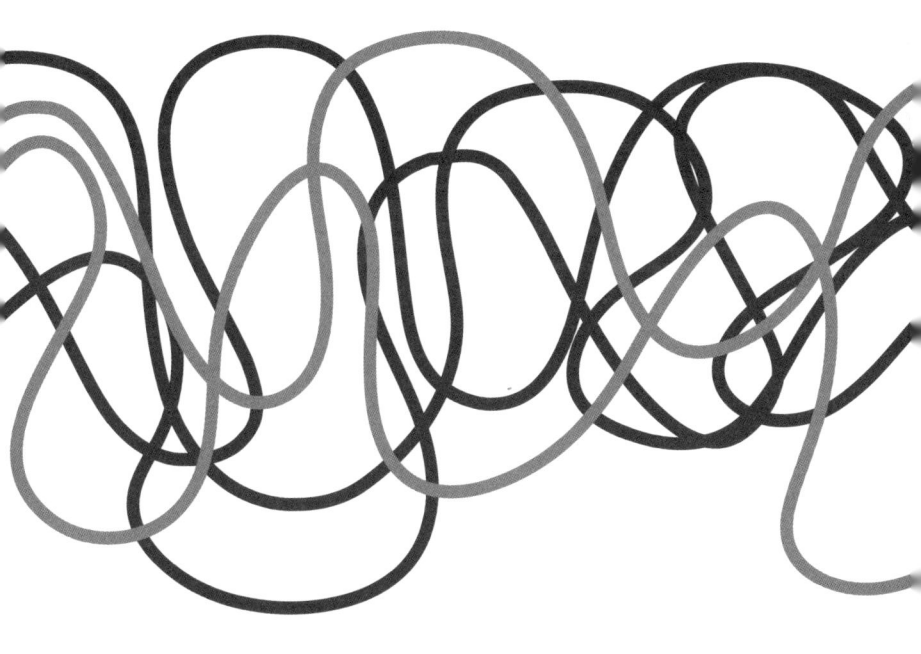

Naoise Dolan is an Irish writer who has published two novels, *Exciting Times* (2020) and *The Happy Couple* (2023). Her work has been shortlisted and longlisted for prizes including the Women's Prize, the Dylan Thomas Prize and the Polari Prize.

Life as a Second Language

When I started studying Japanese aged sixteen, I felt accommodated by the level of social explanation and betrayed that I'd never received it before. The textbook explained not only the literal meaning of new phrases but the subtle implicit cues. To say you're not in the mood for something, for instance, you can say it's 'ちょっと...', i.e. 'a bit …'

Irish people also communicate in this elliptical fashion. There are a million gaps where you're supposed to know what to fill in. Nobody ever gave me a textbook. It would have been much simpler if they had.

I am, you see, autistic. I'm also smart. There is nothing I can't understand once it has been clearly explained. Most of these explanations are ones I have had to provide for myself through trial and error.

In any given social situation, I try to be amenable and fair. When I get the response I want (acceptance, warmth), I repeat the behaviour that prompted it. When the feedback is less desirable (indifference, scorn) I try a different approach the next time. Once I have gone through this process, I can explain the pros and cons of different strategies much more lucidly than someone who's never had to break it down. But it feels like I'm always the one doing the work. If only someone else could do it for me and present their findings in a manual.

The closest thing available is etiquette books. These I find addictive: *Where were you all my life?* I wonder as I tear through the pages of each new one. But no text can prepare you for every possible scenario. When I'm forced to freestyle, all bets are off.

So I try to place myself in situations where others will give me the benefit of the doubt. For this reason, I love language-learning.

Not all language textbooks explain social norms as clearly as that Japanese one did in my teens. Where the perceived cultural dissonance is smaller, it's taken for granted that more will be implicitly understood; a French or Italian textbook will tell you the phrases with which you can ask for the bill, but not how to get the waiter's attention. (Incidentally, I once made an Italian friend laugh by asking if it would be sufficient to make '*contatto degli occhi*' with the waiter. It turns out you have to say '*contatto visivo*' for eye contact; '*contatto degli occhi*' makes it sound like the pupils are physically touching. This is indeed how eye contact feels to me with people I don't know well, but I force myself to do it so they won't find me suspicious.)

Textbooks don't solve everything, then. But one thing is always true: when you have a foreign accent, people know you're making a conscious effort to learn rules that don't come naturally to you. They bear that in mind. Sometimes they can still be cruel, especially if they've never learnt a foreign language themselves. But nobody has ever given me as hard a time for my social mistakes in foreign languages as they do for the ones I make in English.

★

Professionally, I write novels and various other bits and bobs. I've published two books and a respectable swathe of short stories, essays and articles. An Italian interviewer once asked me if writing was a hobby or therapy for me; 'È il mio mestiere,' I replied – it's my job. For hobbies/therapy, I look elsewhere: I draw, play piano, learn languages.

I speak six languages – English, French, German, Irish, Italian and Spanish – though my abilities fluctuate depending on which of them I've been using most recently. I also know some Japanese, Cantonese and Mandarin from having studied them at certain points. Last year I started learning Russian, but got invited soon afterwards to two literary festivals in Romania and Slovakia – so now I have switched to Romanian and Slovak, at least until the festivals are behind me. I always learn at least the basic phrases before I go abroad. It's not a monastic sacrifice, a tourist's tithe; it's half the fun of travel for me. I feel free speaking other languages in a way I never really do in English.

Since I have a native speaker's accent in English – albeit one that's hard to place, a bit of my parents' rural Irish accents, a bit of Dublin, a bit of London – I am expected to know the rules. When I break them, people assume it's out of malice. There's more latitude when I speak a foreign language: my accent makes it clear that I'm trying my best. If I'm blunt, people assume it's because I didn't have the right vocabulary to be subtle.

I meet many people who tell me they're scared of speaking foreign languages. They ask where I find my confidence. The honest answer is that I don't – I'm just yet more terrified in English. I feel no shame when I say the wrong thing in Italian. That I'm speaking it at all is a miracle; it's a language I taught myself in a few months without taking classes or living in the country. There is just as valid a contextual explanation for my social missteps in English – I'm autistic – but this one isn't as widely understood.

In school I loved grammar. Like most anglophones, I didn't learn much of it in the classroom, but I devoured it in library books at home. I obsessed over punctuation and changing trends: the decline of the subjunctive, the gradual Americanisation of Irish and British English. Suddenly the rules of communication could be explicitly studied and debated. For me it was much less daunting to read hundreds of pages about grammar than to try to sound normal in the playground, where I spoke too formally and couldn't understand slang. 'Normal' was a dialect with no visible governing structures. I couldn't find a conjugation table for normal, nor a vocabulary list nor a summary of scholars' views. You were normal or you weren't, and I wasn't. Grammar, though, I could work on. Grammar, I could learn.

Learning how our language has mutated over history is therapeutic for me: there's less shame in bungling modern communication once you realise how changeable it is. It's not an innate and eternal truth; it's just how we happen to do things right now. Take the trajectory of the second-person pronoun, which in today's English is always 'you'. We used to have more options: thou/thee for a single person, you/ye for plural. Over time, you/ye began doing double service as a singular formal pronoun, rather like '*vous*' in French or the royal 'we'; one person could be 'you' if they were important enough. Over time it became impolite to call anyone 'thou/thee', and these forms – along with the case differentiation marked by 'ye' – disappeared almost entirely.

Traces of these distinctions do remain. My grandmother, a lifelong Leitrimer, said 'ye' to indicate plural-you until she died in 2010. The Dublin English I grew up speaking made abundant use of the plural 'youse' and 'yiz', while the American 'y'all' does a similar job. Thou/thee still appear in some Lancashire and Black Country British dialects, and lines like 'Thee shut thi mouth' surface throughout Yorkshire writer Barry Hines's 1968 novel *A Kestrel for a Knave*. I love these traces, these clues that tell you not only who a person is but whom they feel close to. So much of social in- and out-groups are invisible to me: as a child and teenager I was never sure when I was allowed to consider anyone my friend, let alone understand why X person wouldn't talk to Y person. When I find a language-based snippet of evidence – 'If they're an Irish person who still says ye, maybe they identify with a community similar to my grandmother's' – it's like donning goggles that allow me to momentarily see the lines of allegiance that everyone else does.

My interest in language is descriptive, not prescriptive. I have no desire to tell people how to talk: I just listen when they do, then ask myself why they said it the way they did. Still, I can't help having a soft spot for history's most prominent thou-defenders, the Quakers. They fought a losing battle to resist linguistic change because they disliked how formal 'you' calcified social rank. (There is nothing my autistic soul loves more than losing battles.) Now that we all 'you' each other, the pronoun no longer demarcates clout – but when thou was still in currency, the you/thou distinction reinforced the class system. In a 1671 pamphlet,

Wired Our Own Way

founding member of the Quakers George Fox described the usages of his time like this: '[F]or amongst the great and rich ones of the Earth, they will either thou or you one another if they be [equal] in degree, as they call it; but if a man of low degree in the Earth come to speak to any of them, then he must you the rich man, but the rich man will thou him.' A decade earlier Fox had written a whole book arguing to 'thou' everyone: *A Battle-Door for Teachers & Professors to Learn Singular & Plural; You to Many, and Thou to One: Singular One, Thou; Plural Many, You*, published in 1660.

Over the following few centuries, the Quakers remained thou-proponents. 'Supposing it be the captain of the Pequod, what dost thou want of him?' demands a Quaker in Herman Melville's 1851 novel *Moby-Dick*. (Like many modern English-speakers, Melville's narrator associates thee and thou not with plain speech but with a 'stately dramatic … idiom'.) Even as late as the twenty-first century, an American Quaker Plain Speech manual last revised in 2003 says that the form is still in use but its conjugation has mutated with the times: 'speakers have naturally become less "proficient" as the forms have begun to die out. Also, some Quakers now are less careful in distinguishing plural from singular, using "thee" even to more than one person.' The manual later says that '[n]early all European languages share [an] association of plurality and deference'. (But not, incidentally, Irish, which makes a singular/plural distinction of *tú/sibh* but has no separate formal 'you'.)

Much of thou's decline has to do with social status becoming more fluid. The industrial revolution and the rise of the middle class brought greater uncertainty over which pronoun to use, and 'you' was the one less likely to give offence. When enough people are socially anxious, it can change an entire language.

In other European languages I still find this you-business a treacherous tightrope. Informal-you can be overfamiliar, while formal-you can imply that you want to maintain a cold distance or that you think they're old. In German and French I default to formal-you, while in Italian and Spanish informal-you is my go-to. (In Spanish, though, it varies by country; when I was in Mexico last year at the Guadalajara book fair, I heard the formal '*usted*' more often than I do in Spain. You can give yourself a bespoke hernia trying to keep your *ustede*s and *vosotro*s and *vo*s and *tú* straight, depending where on you are.)

Confusing as the you-malarkey can be, I feel the same tingle reading up on it that I do when I research English grammar. The lack of a manual for human contact in my childhood was so daunting that any social instruction, any at all, now makes me feel held.

The disappearance of the thou/you distinction in English doesn't mean we've lost layers of formality. As a modern-day practitioner, I'm often stumped by questions of tone that are far harder than the 'you' stuff to just google. I need thirty minutes to respond to a professional email: two seconds to type my actual answer, and twenty-eight minutes fifty-eight seconds to agonise over how to add the right filler phrases. *As I said in my last email* can be a declaration of war; *Thanks in advance!*, complete with exclamation mark, can indicate that you want the person's head on a spit.

That's not to say anglophones are uniquely passive-aggressive. Germans are well able to give us a run for our money. Their reputed national directness hasn't prevented my neighbours from leaving all manner of anonymous notes on one another's doors. (I have yet to receive one, but I await the day with all due trepidation.) In Italy I have made a number of sartorial gaffes because nobody would respond clearly when I asked what to wear; they assumed I didn't need it spelled out that my black Uniqlo turtleneck with a hole in one of the elbows wasn't quite the thing for a classical concert in June. I face similar problems on the British literary scene. You ask what to wear to an award ceremony, they say to go in whatever you're most comfortable in, and when you show up it just so happens that everyone else felt most comfortable in identical outfits that are nothing like yours.

For such social questions – which I pose to others with the wild-eyed desperation of one who's been burnt before – there clearly is an established answer that nearly everyone knows. ('Nearly everyone' because I don't.) So why don't people simply share that answer when asked? The thinking, I gather, is that it's insulting to tell an adult things that any child should grasp.

Ah, but I don't grasp it. This difference between me and people who intuitively understand social norms does not go away from pretending it doesn't exist. If you just give me the information, I can make my own choice about what to do with it. Maybe I'll still wear something different. But if I want to blend in, I'll have the option. I do often figure things out for myself eventually, but it's a lot of work. I wish I didn't have to keep reinventing the wheel.

★

Language-learning feeds into my writing. I write mainly in English, but learning other languages deepens my understanding of the one I work in. The peculiarities of English are laid bare when you find out how other languages phrase things; you scrutinise each idiom, each cliché. There's a loss of innocence, and with it an acquisition of power. English is no longer all-encompassing when you've read outside it, dreamt outside it, lived outside it.

As an exercise, I write the odd scrap of fiction in other languages, but I think it's unlikely I'd ever publish any of it. I can be correct in other languages, but correctness isn't enough; to write good fiction, I need to be able to break the rules. And contrary to all canned wisdom, knowing the rules isn't enough to break them. It's necessary, but it's not sufficient. You also need to know whether you're breaking them in a way that works, and this requires a level of proficiency that goes far beyond mere communication.

The sort of English I'm interested in writing holds each sentence to tight account. I need to be happy that each word is not only adequate, but the best word I could possibly use. This scrutiny never ceases; I can't stand to read anything I've published more than a month ago because the fresh eye always reveals more words I want to change, and now can't. (For this reason I dislike reading aloud from my work. My honest answer when asked if I'd like to do a reading at events is: 'It will be unpleasant for me, but if people would really enjoy it then on balance it's worthwhile.' But this frank cost/benefit analysis can sound to neurotypicals like a veiled way of saying that I hate them and their request, so I usually just say: 'Yes, sure.' They're not really asking if I'd *like to* read, after all; they're asking if I insuperably object to doing it, which I don't.)

If I stopped making progress in English, stopped finding new and satisfying ways to break the rules, then I'd turn to other languages to feel that thrill of discovery. But for now, at least, I'm still finding new things I can do every time I sit down to write. Having other options makes me more convinced that English is a good fit and not just a default.

Still, I find other uses for the languages. I've done literary events conducted entirely in German and Italian and I'll be doing one in Spanish this Halloween. I journal in whichever language I feel rustiest in – French at the moment – and I enjoy being able to keep up with new non-anglophone fiction. Even when I can't read the original language, it's often easier to find a book translated into German than into English; Germans read much more widely in translation than anglophones do, so learning German has given me a ticket to many other literary scenes.

I've had entire relationships, both professional and personal, that have only ever been conducted in a foreign language. These connections are special: I embody a different side of myself that people who only speak English are quite literally unable to understand. Each language comes with its own associated set of experiences. My personality is different in each of them, though somehow it's all ultimately me.

The social manual I craved as a teenager doesn't seem to be forthcoming anytime soon. But language-learning has given me something better: self-forgiveness. More often than not when I speak a foreign language, my blunders are met with kindness. The odd time that I encounter impatience, I simply remind myself that how others treat me is a reflection of them, not me. *They're being quite rude*, I think, or *Wow, that was weird* – simple thoughts, but ones I have to remind myself how to think, because my reigning assumption throughout my childhood and adolescence was that any social discord was my fault. Now that's changed. I'm proud of my accent and even of my mistakes; they show that my environment didn't just hand me the language, that I've learnt it the hard way. And ultimately, when I'm the one doing the accommodating – when I'm playing on hard mode so that the other person can stay in easy mode – who cares if they can tell that their language isn't natively mine?

I carry over this new approach when I return to English. Most neurotypicals have no idea how much effort I'm making, how well I'm doing if you account for the fact that I have taught myself every last thing. Maybe they'll never know how much work goes into it. But I know, and that's enough.

Colm Brady, Dublin-born, is a graduate of fine art from the Dublin Institute of Technology and the National College of Art and Design. He lives and works as a fine artist in West Cork with his partner of nine years.

Makeshift Oasis

Having been identified as being on the autism spectrum in 2023 at the age of fifty-five was no great revelation. The assessment with a clinical psychologist was a logical step forward after decades of internal dialogue. During the assessment I felt like I was, quite gently, being diagnosed as myself. There was little introduced to me in that process that I hadn't previously recognised. Being mildly aged as I am, it wasn't so much predicting a future as acknowledging a past. My life could now be reviewed through a new lens.

One might ask, 'Why would you want an autism assessment later in life?' Well, I doubt very much that any adult would be doing it in the pursuit of novelty. The majority will have lived with an awareness that they have struggled in areas of life that their peers did not. For instance, I struggle with an inability to filter and prioritise my attention on sounds in my environment. I hear everything at the same level. My day-to-day life would include less adrenaline if I didn't have constant incoming audio data. For example, those who choose not to wear headphones while listening to their devices, the clicking of phone keys, the clattering of cutlery, and perhaps the most irritating, the sound of snack packaging rustling in the cinema. It was a revelation to realise I was experiencing misophonia, a physical and emotional fight-or-flight response to everyday sounds that, prior to last year, I'd never heard of. I had toddled along with daily discomfort, oftentimes avoiding various social situations such as public transport, noisy restaurants and cinemas. Surely, everyone must hear these annoying sounds and the bigger question was, how do they cope? It hadn't crossed my mind that others didn't experience similar issues or negative effects from everyday sounds.

My childhood was solitary. I hadn't developed friendships. My attempts didn't yield positive results. In regards to daily social interaction, an early experience on a primary-school day trip to the RDS in 1977 illustrates a clear difference in what I perceived as normal social behaviour relative to my peer group. The coach deposited my class, everyone donning navy and grey uniforms, outside the exhibition buildings. Inside the building we sounded like a noisy penguin colony moving on fast forward, all dispersed around the exhibition stalls in previously formed cliques. Not being part of any clique myself, I awkwardly trailed Damien and Des, two classmates whom I felt to be outsiders. Des was the shortest kid in our year, blond and usually cranky. Damien was dark, witty and a tad highly strung. I tagged along, hoping to find myself part of a little group until Des turned to look at me, rolling his eyes, and said, 'Goodbye Colm!' They scuttled quickly around a corner. I didn't follow. I wandered alone around the stalls until it was time to meet outside at the coach and return to the school.

I always felt kids my age possessed a script I wasn't given. They were quick and intuitive. I often wondered at what point I was supposed to join in and, more importantly, what to say. I would usually look for a moment to introduce pedigree dogs into the conversation. A subject I had obsessed about for years. The enthusiasm with which

I delivered the information was combined with my having a stammer. It rarely went well. I mistakenly thought they would be as interested as I was in an interesting subject. Isn't everybody interested in dogs?

A year later, to my delight, I had managed to befriend another dog-lover, Mrs Mink, who lived nearby. Her house wasn't far and I could visit for a few hours every few weeks. She had five Japanese Chins (a breed of dog, not a physical attribute). Pretty little black and white dogs that skipped along the arms of her sofas tilting their heads in wide-eyed wonder like little marmoset monkeys. I never once heard them bark, which I attributed to their primate status. I didn't know Mrs Mink's age at that time. I was eleven, which placed her, in my eyes, somewhere between forty and seventy-five. Regardless of the time of day, she would slowly sip what I assumed was 'cola' from a small glass as we chatted on about pedigree dogs. Most days her words would begin to slur a little as my visit went on and the glass was topped up. For reasons I can only surmise, my mother wasn't happy with me visiting Mrs Mink. So much so, she suggested karate lessons as an alternative. This was a pretty drastic step for my mother considering I was born with bilateral clubbed feet. I had corrective surgery as an infant and was able to walk well but running was an issue. My balance could be off and the flexibility of my feet was very limited. My mom's letters to school excusing me from gym and sports didn't tally with her suddenly suggesting I take up karate. I resisted, and in the end, I didn't do karate. I held fast to my dog obsession.

Age sixteen was a watershed year for me. I began speech therapy at a child guidance clinic. The biology teacher at school had approached me one day after class and broached the topic of my stammer. She told me she had grown up with a stammer and had attended a speech therapist to help resolve it. It was so nice to have somebody discuss it with me. The other teachers hadn't mentioned it. At home it had been mainly ignored or might have elicited an occasional 'try to speak properly' comment. Attending the speech therapist showed there wasn't a physical cause for my stammer. I had been a chatterbox from an early age, apparently enjoying my vocabulary. The psychologist on the team suggested there were emotional factors behind it.

At that time, I made the decision to write a letter to my mother acknowledging my sexuality. What motivated the decision I don't recall, nonetheless, it didn't go down well. My parents died four months apart in my final year of secondary school. My mother from a heart attack and my father from cancer. The family home was sold by my elder siblings. The following years of my late teens were very difficult. My fledging into what is seen as conventional functioning amounted to a series of stumbles. I hadn't learnt domestic skills or time management; how to be the administrator of my life was entirely new. Other people my age seemed to be intuitively moving into adulthood. I was an unrecognised autistic teenager finding his way (the good old, bad old days of not having a clue). As a result, any of my nostalgia for the 1980s is entirely limited to the music. Struggles occurred as I went along, leading to brief periods of counselling. Looking back, I now realise the therapists were not familiar with what we know today as neurodiversity. Therapy focused on family dynamics rather than noticing and exploring differences in how I experience the world, for example the rhythm of my executive functioning, my sensory issues, my burnouts leading to social withdrawal. This wasn't raised at the time.

Being gay was something I had leaned on for years as an explanation for my feeling different. I told myself I would find a gay community after school and instantly feel connection. I went along to a youth group meeting in Dublin when I was twenty-one. Derek, the group facilitator (was that even a word in the Ireland of 1988?), found it acceptable to declare, 'Colm! You are weird!' I suppose back then a person organising a youth group was just required to have a key to the door and a kettle for the tea break. Charm was entirely optional. I was able to shake that off, although it has obviously stuck with me. As is often the case with the Dereks of this world, they assume their words are a revelation to you: Derek, with a mere three word, had joined a queue of others over the years. And like my schooldays, another disheartening attempt at fitting in had once again failed. I stayed the course, however, and this time something was different. The group had about fifteen people attending. There were two or three quirky guys that engaged me in conversation. We quickly recognised something in each other that placed us on the periphery of a group that was already a minority. Derek may have been the latest Damien and Des all grown up, but I suddenly had my little makeshift crew, and for the first time I felt I had a friend or two. In retrospect, it was obvious we had our traumas. Several of us had been raised with a level of reticence in our various families of origin that, at the very least, led to estrangement, often leaving us feeling uncomfortable at family events and gatherings. Intuitively, there was an understanding between us that we were outsiders and hadn't been 'figured out'.

Having friends was a new experience for me. My many quirks were accepted and matched by the eccentricities of my new friends, and their journeys resonated with me. There was little judgement and when we laughed we laughed with each other rather than at each other. Although there were those who would step away from our inner circle from time to time to find their tribe elsewhere, the basic group remained intact. I suppose if I supported and justified myself during my isolation in my youth by being aware of my sexuality, I could continue to process my many differences until I was ready to identify neurodivergence. The wait would be a long one, however.

I was accepted to art college in the 1990s and it was a turning point. It was as if the outsiders had congregated in a cradle that celebrated diversity. I confidently welcomed the 'you think differently' and 'you're a bit different, aren't you?' comments from those more polite than the Dereks and Deses. Thinking outside the box, or simply not recognising the box at all, was beneficial in pursuing creativity. 'Top down thinking,' seeing the bigger picture first, may be useful in some professions, but 'bottom up' or sometimes 'sideways' thinking, and being captivated by and investigating the details, is more important to success in the arts and sciences. I find that creativity is a comfortable place for me to be. I don't consider it a luxury as it simply feels familiar. I'm more at ease in those processes: it is a place to breathe, where the unexpected is always around the corner if you are open to it. Being neurodivergent has given me a road map to follow my perception of the world and I feel lucky to frequently look and wonder. For those who ask, 'Why would you want a label?' – well, in all likelihood, we've already had many unpleasant labels from the school playground over the years. There will always be a Des or a Derek. They can move back to their comfort zones as we should be free to move towards ours. Discovering, on our own terms and in our own time, why we tick and naming it, doesn't compare.

I may have always felt like an outsider but after all these years I'm OK with that. It has given me my life and my love for the people I share it with. I am neurodivergent, I don't have neurodivergence any more than a neurotypical person has neurotypicality. Although my revelation came in my fifties, it's filled in the gaps in my understanding of my journey, and most importantly, tells me to celebrate the fact that I made it this far.

Freya von Noorden Pierce is a creative copywriter, living and working in Amsterdam since 2015. She sporadically writes about whatever comes into her head on her website, **fraeji.com**.

The Canary

There is a piece of writing by e.e. cummings where he says, 'To be nobody-but-yourself – in a world which is doing its best, night and day, to make you everybody else – means to fight the hardest battle which any human being can fight; and never stop fighting.'

In this literary instance, I know he is referring to the life of a poet – indeed, the title of this piece is 'A Poet's Advice'. However, when my partner showed me the excerpt in his book, I felt it applied to something else, and thus I write it here.

I've been on a road to forgiveness of some sort. For a large portion of my life, certainly since I was small, I've felt like I've been on some sort of test run. As if I've not really been present throughout my days and that, at some point in the future, everything would simply click into place – the video of my life would suddenly come into focus after buffering away for years. This isn't to say that I haven't felt joy, anger, euphoria or any other emotion during that time. In fact, I've felt them in abundance. I just couldn't grapple with why I felt them so intently, when the smallest thing – a delayed train or a sudden noise – would send me into a spiral, much to the bemusement or concern of those around me.

I've learnt this is called dissociation, that fog-like haze you might feel when your brain goes into overload. In certain dissociative states I can float above myself, looking down at the room I'm in; a kind of lucid dreaming.

They say trauma starts in childhood, so here's a story. I remember my teachers in primary school, exasperated, asking me why I didn't want to play with the other children, not understanding that I just wanted to immerse myself in my intricately detailed make-believe cocoon, all by myself, or hauling me during a fire drill out of a toy box where I'd hidden for hours. I just wanted to remain in my safe little world, where I could make up my own stories and see things in a way that I understood. Sometimes, as an adult, I still revert to this.

And then I think of teenage Freya at senior school who, despite a close-knit and loving friend group and solid academic success, despised every fibre of her being; who was unable to understand why she felt so vastly different from her peers and experienced a creeping dread in every social situation; who wanted to cry in frustration when she couldn't grasp a mathematical problem, picked at her skin or pulled out her hair during exam periods in an attempt to soothe the pressure inside her head.

I remember going to my GP in my first year of university, tearfully begging to be referred to a therapist after weeks of panic attacks and skin-picking – only to be handed a leaflet about meditation and a printout of a list of therapists I could try calling, but 'they probably wouldn't take me' as I wasn't Dutch. My GP told me to try yoga and be grateful that it was 'all in my head' and not in real life.

But now, when I think about that little girl who just wanted to be alone, who was scared of loud noises and couldn't understand the games the other children were playing, I feel my heart swell with sympathy instead of embarrassment and resentment.

It's taken years, but I'm getting there.

I've learnt that this world is not built for neurodivergent people, as much as corporate diversity and inclusion committees may have you believe. The e.e. cummings quote at the beginning of this piece is a good reminder of this. Because in a world that constantly pressures you to fit in, to *play the game* and *get on with things*, those with differing brains suffer. I read that up to 85 per cent of neurodivergent adults are unemployed, and that most studies on autism are carried out on white, European, teenage boys. Most women who are diagnosed autistic spend years suffering with depression and anxiety, and are often brushed off as just *being emotional* until they are finally diagnosed in their late twenties. As a white woman who is only now being able to access these vital health services, I cannot imagine the pain and systemic ignorance towards non-white men and women going through similar battles with their own neurodivergence journeys. While learning about your neurodivergence can be liberating and healing, it's also an exhausting, expensive and time-consuming journey. It shouldn't have to be.

People might say that neurodivergence is a gift, and in some instances, I'm inclined to agree. I'm able to enjoy music and art to an ecstatic degree, recanting riffs and details from songs and books that I read years ago. I'm creative and can go into extreme detail about subjects I'm interested in, sometimes to the annoyance of others – but let me live. After all, who doesn't want to know my bizarre expertise on shows like *Arrested Development*? I'm a good listener and love helping people with their problems, even if I can't reciprocate in the same way with my own. I quickly pick up on people's emotions – my mum calls me a canary in a coal mine – and can be empathetic to a fault.

But there are times when it cripples me, and when it comes with not-so-quirky traits. Certain social situations can absolutely drain me, especially if I'm with large groups of strangers having multiple conversations at once. I physically recoil when people who aren't my closest friends touch me, which can lead to odd looks. When I feel unwell, my anxiety takes over, and I find myself needing to call in sick from work not for physical but for mental stress. When I become overstimulated around others I shut down, often experiencing mutism, and can come off as rude and snappy. I sometimes have to bail on friends and then make action-packed plans to dampen the overwhelming guilt. I'm lucky that my closest friends understand this about me and won't judge, but it doesn't make it any easier. I often feel like I've aged a lot in the last few years, opting to spend my weekends in a low-key manner and going to bed early. I understand this is what I need to do for my body and brain, but I'd have liked to be a bit more rock-and-roll in my twenties. That's just something I have to accept, and ultimately, it's OK.

The world may not be made for us, but you can make it work for you. In fact, demand that it does. Ask for accommodations at work if you need them, and confide in your closest friends when you're struggling. You don't have to be an activist for neurodiversity, but learn to advocate for yourself. Most people's ideas of autism are outdated and archaic, often unintentionally, so encourage those around you to listen. And at the end of the day, telling people your brain works differently doesn't change much, but it'll give you a sense of freedom and safety. Your real friends will take that on board and be your buffer, your security, your protectors, as you are for them.

The rest of the e.e. cummings quote goes:

'Does this sound dismal? It isn't.

It's the most wonderful life on earth.

Or so I feel.'

I think I can relate, to some extent.

This essay has been published anonymously.

Co-Regulating Chaos

'I'm an autistic mom,' I say.

Heads nod with seeming comprehension. 'Oh, your kids are on the spectrum? I'd never have guessed, they look so normal!'

I cringe.

Firstly, because what do they expect my kids to look like, carrots? But secondly, because that's not what I meant. Yes, my kids are autistic, all four of them. But I was trying to tell you that I am too. I was autistic before they were. Now I have to try and explain again that no, I mean me. I am autistic.

Few people ever think of the autistic parent, and yet with the way it often runs in families, support services and the wider public should spare a thought for us, the autistic moms and dads struggling to support our precious kids. I'm about to dish the dirt on some of the serious challenges we face, so let me assure you first that obviously I adore my kids. They are the best part of my life and I cherish each and every one, even when they're being their often-challenging, mischievous selves.

But let's talk about supporting them the way I *know* they need. Let's say they are overwhelmed from the sensory stimuli around them. My middle child is going into shutdown because the place is too noisy and crowded for her. She needs Mom to be on top of it, to recognise it early, remove her from the situation, help her regulate, and then decide whether it is better to return to it or call it a day. But the noisy crowded situation is playing *havoc* with my own tolerances! I can barely focus on the situation, but I have to be 100 per cent for her.

Or my youngest is struggling because the lighting is too overstimulating. She needs something to fidget with to draw her eyes down to her hands and help her settle again. But the lights are making me dizzy myself. Another child is struggling with the changes of plans when a day goes awry. I have to calm them, help them accept the changes and reorient themselves to a new day plan. But I'm feeling all wrong and out of sorts myself because I had a PLAN. And my wonderful, organised, fun plan has been changed and that *wasn't* the plan! I'm reeling and trying to adapt myself.

Professionals often talk about co-regulation. It's a great word. I use it myself. My kid is in a meltdown before bed? I pull them into my arms, talk calmly, reassuringly, and recognise their feelings. Then we work through them together and settle, until all is well with the world again. I feel like a pro. Best parent ever.

The next day we're out at a shop. The radio is on and it's grating at my ears. The place is busy, and the kids are starting to feel it. The two younger ones are bickering. I had PLANNED to go to the playground on the way home, but I just got a call that we have to hurry home earlier than expected. Now the kids will not have their oh-so-necessary climb and swing, so they'll be awful to get to bed. One of them starts wailing about something, but what's really wrong is they need their mom to co-regulate. How? How do I co-regulate them when I'm overwhelmed with noise and change? I try, I do my best, but it feels like it is never enough and my own energy and tolerance plummets even more …

Then one of them needs the bathroom. I never use a hand dryer for myself, nasty noisy things they are. But now bathroom trips involve me gritting my teeth while I cover first one child's then the other's ears while THEY dry their hands. Doesn't seem fair, but then I don't want them to be scared of the damn things like they used to be, so one suffers on.

And it's not just during outings things go wrong. Dinner time is intensely awkward. Each child has their own picky eating habits. Some are all about the taste, some about the texture, some both. One has issues with the way hot food smells. But I'm quite picky myself! So every dinner, by necessity, consists of five different, specially prepared meals – of which, on average, two to three will not be eaten anyway, even though I was ill just looking at the texture of one of them cooking.

But let's say you are the kind of autistic who thrives on sensory input. Never get overwhelmed by it. What about social situations? I love social situations with my friends. Planned ones, doing things I like, with people I like, and with planned recovery time after. I do NOT like social settings with strangers. I struggle to remember names, faces and connections. This makes dealing with other parents in relation to school and extra-curriculars a special kind of hell! Someone says hello at the school gate like they know me? How do they know me? Whose parent are they? Which of my kids are they asking about? School collection time is like entering a minefield every day, never knowing who you'll meet, or who they are when you DO meet them.

And playdates? Of course my child needs playdates. They need the social connection with their peers, the fun … But that means I need to identify and engage with a parent to arrange these things, and then often talk with the parent extensively on the day too. Playdates are exhausting! What does one talk about in this situation? Who should one talk with about it? Am I oversharing? Every minute detail of the interactions needs to be analysed behind the mask to try and put your child's best foot forward, to not sabotage their chances with this parent's kid …

This constant theme of working through my own discomforts, co-regulating when I'm overwhelmed and giving my all when there is nothing left to give is common for us autistic parents. And it has follow-on effects that few may have thought of.

Let's talk special interests. I have them, of course I do. I love them. Diving into them helps me regulate myself and ground myself. But at 11 p.m. at night, when I'm barely holding myself together after hours and hours of trying everything under the sun to get them to sleep, and the last child finally drifts off, am I able to start into enjoying them? Rarely. So I don't get to experience the soothing balm they offer, and I'm not particularly regulated in the morning when it all starts again.

In fact, since I had children, I struggle to even start a new TV series or book series. It's not because of a lack of time, although that is obviously another issue, but because of the emotional investment my autistic brain needs to allow it to begin something new, something unknown. I just don't have that energy to invest.

So I've been complaining and pointing out all the problems inherent with the familial nature of autism.

Would it surprise you to know that I find a lot of benefits too?

When I'm totally done with a busy environment, my child often is too. We can escape together.

'Mom I want to go home. I don't like the noise.'

'You and me both, buddy!'

And when I have to squint through the busy lights indoors, it's a quick early warning that some of my kids are going to find this particular lighting a bit much, and I should act accordingly.

When the time comes to explain their autism to them, it's easy. I get it, and I can talk about myself and how we're alike. They're not different or strange, they're just like Mom.

My own lifelong experience with being autistic has given me a perspective that I feel has really helped my parenting. Unlike what seems like the majority of autistic parents my own age, I knew I was autistic before I had children. I had plenty of time to learn about it and process it before I ever became pregnant, and was able to watch them grow up knowing there was a chance each of them would be like me. When their development veered away from what would be considered typical, it was never a cause for concern, just another trait to note for later and cause for a knowing nod. I was able to get them diagnosed nice and early, even though they were fierce maskers, and get them the support they needed from the start.

My similar perspective also helps in making decisions for them. One child wants desperately to play a certain sport, but finds every training session overwhelming and therefore is unable to participate on match days. We persevere for years in spite of the difficulty because it's what they want. I remember wanting things that were difficult for me. We make adaptations, throw energy and patience into it, ignore the many long trips where the child ended up not playing … Now, as a teenager, it's one of the most regulating parts of their week. A small victory for me as a parent.

Another time, my younger child wants to leave a party. They're not having fun anymore and are just over the whole social environment. Do I keep them there so they don't stand out like a sore thumb? Or do I bring them away as soon as they find it overwhelming? I decide to take them home. I remember what it was like when social settings got too much as a kid. There'll be no benefits to them from pushing it.

Of course there are wrong calls too.

'This is delicious!' announces one child, trying chocolate mousse for the first time from a grandparent's plate.

'What do you mean delicious, how can you even stand that awful texture?' I demand, having lovingly sheltered them from the evil substance for years already.

As the kids grow into teens, we can joke about our autism together. We share funny memes about it, as if we're part of a secret club with so many other people across the world, and we understand each other. When things get harder in teenage years, and they have problems I can't fix, I can empathise and share similar stories from my youth. My worry for them about the big-kid things I can't fix so easily becomes harder and harder, more and more draining.

Do I look forward to a time when I again have the mental energy to pick up a new book and read it, or try out a new TV show? When I can indulge my interests to my heart's content? Of course I do. I yearn for it desperately. But knowing it probably will not happen until my house is quiet, and my kids are grown, I also dread it. I want to savour each and every year with them, enjoy every little moment. Until then I'll just have to run on their hugs and chocolate.

Jennifer Poyntz is an Irish writer and PhD researcher. Through her work at Trinity College Dublin, Jennifer strives to help disabled students feel empowered in their education. Jennifer writes and speaks about her experiences of being autistic and living with two chronic illnesses: Ehlers-Danlos Syndrome (hypermobility sub-type) and secondary Addison's disease.

The Tin Man's Heart

Let me paint you two parallel pictures.

Imagine, if you can, a young woman. Her hair is a cross between blonde and brunette and, though it is not yet noticeable, thinning rapidly. Her face is adorned with freckles that are neither a constellation nor a smattering, but rather an army. They stand out like hole punches against her pallid skin. This young woman wears baby-pink Doc Martens, a sundress patterned with daisies and a second-hand cardigan from Oxfam with fraying sleeves.

She is eighteen years old.

Now, please imagine another young woman. In truth, the same young woman. She is no longer pale, but translucent, with bluish circles under her eyes. Her lips are permanently dry, cracked and bleeding. This young woman wears grey biker shorts and an oversized Harvard sweater. Penneys' best. There is a toothpaste stain above her right collarbone. Her hair, now the texture of straw, resembles a bird's nest atop her head, but still holds some vestiges of summer sunlight.

This young woman is now twenty-eight years old. And she is *tired*.

Her name is Jen. Jennifer for work, Jens by her dad's side of the family and JenJen by her one, beloved sister.

Eighteen-year-old Jen sits with her mom in the waiting room of her GP and has the energy to consider whether it is embarrassing to have one's mother come into the doctor's office. Still, Young Jen is not yet adept at manoeuvring medical staff alone. She sits with her hands under her thighs as the tinny music from Radio Kerry pierces her pores. Still, when another patient, a lady with hair the colour of steel wool, catches sight of Young Jen and watches her thumb through a *National Geographic* from 1998, Jen is sure to make eye contact. She constructs a smile that stretches to her eyes. Eighteen-year-old Jen gives the people what they want.

Twenty-eight-year-old Jen sits in the GP waiting room alone, legs outstretched, and ankles crossed. A woman nearby nurses her sick baby. Whooping cough, maybe. To her right, an old man who smells vaguely of whiskey and cow shit tries to make eye contact with her. Older Jen would rather die than talk to another human being and so, she doesn't.

Both Jens hear the doctor approaching before she opens the waiting room door. Dr Jane observes Young Jen with enthused, empathetic generosity, and Older Jen with the energy of a wilting sunflower. Young Jen smiles benignly and allows her mom to walk through the door first. Older Jen raises an eyebrow and gets to her feet before saying:

'I know, Jane, your favourite patient is back – try to contain your excitement.'

Dr Jane's office smells much the same to both Older and Young Jen. Latex and the faint mildewy scent of the damp cardboard overflowing from the recycling bin beyond the open window. The walls are a sage-green shade in both memories, though the latter timeline has added a few more unnerving mosaics of various species of fish in beechwood frames.

When Dr Jane takes her seat, she turns towards the Jens with a wide smile.

'So, what can I do for you?' Dr Jane asks, slapping her thighs lightly, indicating that she is ready to get to work.

Young Jen blushes. She is nervous – not yet a veteran in this game of chronic illness cat and mouse.

'I have a really sore throat. Like I feel as though it's on fire,' Young Jen explains, wincing over her words.

Her mother takes over then, explaining that Jen had already missed two weeks of school and considering that she is in Leaving Cert year, she is concerned. 'Another round of antibiotics, perhaps,' Jen's mother prompts Dr Jane. After a brief examination of Young Jen's overly sensitive gag reflex, Dr Jane pulls out her prescription pad.

'Do we have to take penicillin?' Young Jen's mother asks with genuine worry. 'It's just that after the first dose of the last round I noted a massive decline in Jen's mood.'

Young Jen nods limply in support. It's true. It hadn't been after the first dose, but rather after the first day, three doses total, when Young Jen had first wanted to kill herself. When Jen's mother had googled it, she'd unearthed only anecdotal evidence of other people finding penicillin impacting their mood and they both know that in the medical sphere anecdotal evidence is as good as no evidence at all.

Dr Jane frowns at this.

'How odd, I've never heard of a reaction like it – but of course, you can take another form of antibiotic.'

A new prescription is drawn up and Young Jen and Not-Yet-Weary Mom are ushered from the room.

Fifty euro, pretty please, says Delia on the front desk.

★

Wired Our Own Way

A decade later, twenty-eight-year-old Jen crosses her legs in Dr Jane's uncomfortable office chair, holding herself tightly. She has things to remember and remembering grows more difficult by the day. The Post-it note in her hand with her precious notes scribbled down is damp with sweat.

'So, what can I do for you?' Dr Jane is a good doctor. Jen has always known this. But sometimes, even that isn't enough.

'Well, as you can imagine, I'm back here because nothing's changed. The endocrinologist found nothing abnormal in my bloodwork and did not think my blood pressure dropping every time I stand was unusual.'

Dr Jane is already turning back to her computer, pulling up the patient report from the private hospital in town. Undeterred, Older Jen continues.

'He actually held his hands up to me and said, "I haven't a rashers!"' Older Jen swallows over her irritation at this. 'So, I'm back here. Same symptoms, no ideas.'

The rest of the appointment went as they all do. Dr Jane asked how much Jen's ill health was impacting her life. Work was becoming near impossible, and she hadn't seen her friends in a long time, if they even still existed. But the antidepressants helped her to get out of bed, so the crisis team didn't need to be called.

The list of symptoms is rehashed.

Dizziness. Rapid heartbeat. Tingly in hands and toes. Dry eyes. Aching joints. Constant thirst. Regular throat infections. Lack of appetite. Persistent headaches, occasionally becoming light-sensitive migraines. Digestive issues. Brain fog. Intermittent ear pain. Hand cramps. Muscle stiffness. Night sweats. Sinus congestion. Constantly swollen glands in neck.

And worst and most debilitating of all, the bone-crushing exhaustion that had long since surpassed tiredness or even fatigue.

It took almost thirty minutes before Dr Jane said what she had likely wanted to upon first sight of Older Jen.

'I think we're at the end of the line here, Jennifer. I don't know what else I can do for you. We might just be looking at bog standard post-viral fatigue from that very first throat infection.'

In that moment, Older Jen's will to live begins to flake away like flecks of rusted paint. If only Dr Jane knew how close Older Jen was to becoming entirely untethered.

'I'm sorry, I truly am.'

And she was. There was no reason to doubt Dr Jane's sincerity. But she had another job she needed Jane to complete before she could allow the overwhelming feeling of helplessness to crush her. Digging in her corduroy messenger bag, Older Jen pulls out the application form for Disability Allowance. Wordlessly, Dr Jane takes the form and begins completing it. *Significant Ongoing Illness*, she writes.

A lump forms in Jen's throat.

'Actually, I was recently assessed for, ah, autism, and yeah, I'm, ah, autistic,' Jen's words are stilted, sounding uncertain when actually, Jen had never been more sure about anything in her entire life. 'I was wondering if you could put that down, too, along with the physical stuff.'

As Dr Jane continues writing, Older Jen's heart grows heavy in her chest. Each beat a glug.

'Oh.'

This simple word is somehow colder than any of the thousands Dr Jane has uttered in the decade preceding.

When Older Jen doesn't speak, Dr Jane looks up from the form.

'You just don't really fit the bill, if you know what I mean.'

If you know what I mean.

There it is again, the smoke signals and morse code of everyone else. Vague in phraseology, but always ready for the gut-punch of honest cruelty. This time, it came in the form of the three words, capitalised in ink, that Dr Jane wrote.

Autism Spectrum Disorder.

Disorder.

When Dr Jane hands Older Jen back the now-completed form, Older Jen takes a breath and shoves a synthetic heart inside of her Tin Man chest, forcing a grateful smile across her face. At twenty-eight, Older Jen still sometimes gives the people what they want.

Older Jen gets to her feet, giving herself a minute to allow the black spots that disrupt her vision to rise and swash away like an inevitable, eroding tide. Her toes tingle as blood floods to her feet.

Older Jen ushers herself from the sage-green, fishy room.

Fifty euro, pretty please, says Delia on the front desk. Older Jen smiles and complies, because, after all, there is nothing else to do.

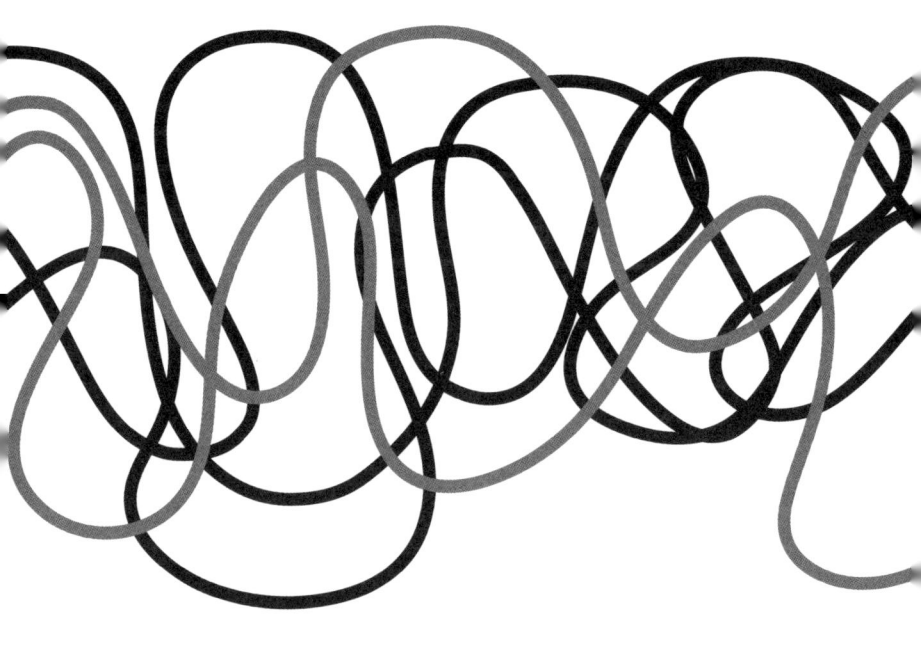

Stefanie Preissner is a writer and actress, best known for creating the TV series *Can't Cope, Won't Cope*. She is the author of books like *Why Can't Everything Just Stay the Same?* and writes a weekly column in the *Sunday Independent LIFE* magazine.

'I don't have a defective version of what you've got'

Me and my brain have been in a battle all my life. I count a lot of things – stairs, cars, the number of times I chew my food – but I cannot count the number of times I have stood in front of a mirror and asked myself, why am I like this?

There's a road I travelled every weekend as a kid – the N20, a road from Mallow to Cork City built with German money through a European investment initiative. It's mostly flat with some inclines but it winds and twists between the villages and hamlets scattered in the County Cork countryside.

Driving towards Mallow, about halfway along, there is a hill on the right. The landscape has changed over the years, but when I was a child there was a forest at the crest of the hill. A bunch of Christmas-type trees gave a jagged and hairy look to the landscape. To the left of the forest there was a single tree, just slightly away from the others. I would quietly contemplate on the journey home whether that tree was leading the pack like a brave warrior with a million soldiers behind, ready to launch. Or perhaps the pack was moving away, trying to put distance between itself and this lone tree?

While my friends were trying to decide which Spice Girl they were or which colour hair mascara to pick, I was thinking about that one tree, on the hill, away from all the others.

I was that tree; close enough to the group to be assumed part of it, but really, when you looked closely, completely disconnected from the masses.

What was wrong with the tree? Was it planted away from the others for a reason? Did it grow that way? Could it ever get back and be part of the group? Eventually, after several years of trying to fit in in my own life, I made a decision about the tree. It wasn't the leader, it wasn't the chosen one, it was indistinguishable but different – just like me.

The tree is long gone, as is the forest. It probably spent a Christmas strangled in tinsel and baubles before being chopped up and burnt. But I'm still here, still close to the group but not fully in it, and I was thirty-four years old before I found out why.

I spent literal decades using myriad nonsense reasons to try to explain me to myself. I knew I needed order and routine. I liked my pencils to be the same height and organised in a line from brightest to darkest. Being on time was as important to me as breathing. I don't like subjectivity. I like what's right to be right and what's wrong to be wrong. I like facts and I never let someone away with a myth. I can be stubborn, and inflexible. Anxiety washes over me when someone changes a plan so I learnt to be rigid, to avoid the distress.

My friends didn't have these traits, so I explained them away by over-identifying with my heritage. *I'm not weird*, I'd reassure myself, *I'm just German*.

Later, once I learnt I was a Taurus, I clung to the zodiac like a life raft. *That's all it is*, I'd reassure myself, *you're a bull*. Then it was introversion, and then personality types, and then it was human design, and then it was birthstones …

Each time I found a new framework for describing people's 'type', I was all over it. 'Please,' I'd beg, 'just give me an explanation!' Turns out the explanation was glaringly clear all along if anyone had been trained enough to look for it. It was never that I was German or Taurean – I was autistic.

I'm autistic right now as I sit in a café writing this article. There's a woman sitting at the window wearing a beanie cap with sequins that catch the sunlight and fling it violently onto the ceiling or the wall depending on the angle of her head. When she looks at her watch the sequins fling the sun into my eyes and I can't see my laptop screen. Why does she need to know the time every three minutes? She's either bored, late, or worried about becoming either of those things.

The coffee machine grinds coffee beans every time someone orders a cup. This shop sells only coffee – why don't they grind up more beans in anticipation of the inevitable orders? It's like they're surprised every time – 'Oh gosh, an Americano? I'll have to grind some beans!' The sound chews up my brain for a few seconds each time it starts, and I have to take a moment to sort myself out and refocus before the next person's order tries to envelop me again.

The banging. Why do baristas have to bang the handle so aggressively? Can't you just tip the old coffee grinds out or use a spatula? Of course, I realise that I'm the problem here. The accommodations needed to make this environment tolerable would be unreasonable for me to request. I gather my things and wander the streets trying to find somewhere to write. Places are too tense, too warm, too much like Limerick Junction or just 'too' anything.

When everything feels too something, it's easy to feel like you're not enough. Eventually, like a failed Goldilocks, I go back home.

It's not that sounds irritate me. It's more like I feel if I keep hearing this noise I will get lost in it. I will lose a sense of where I am and what's happening. Noises can swallow me up and spit me out somewhere other than where I want to be.

Have you ever heard a song on the radio and it fires you back into a memory you were not expecting? After the song finishes, you find you've wandered into a different room or, if you were driving, you have no recollection of the route you took. It's like the song stole you for a few minutes. My experience is like that, but it can be triggered by any sound. So, I block out the noise with headphones or by covering my ears or playing the same things over and over again. It's just me trying to have control of my day.

Having a brain that diverges even slightly from the types of brain that most people have can make you feel like you were born on the wrong planet. The most important thing I'd like to teach people is that a neurodivergent brain is not a malfunctioning neurotypical brain. I don't have a defective version of what you've got.

The reason this is the prevailing thought is because people think that neurotypical reactions, being the most common, are the correct ones. We learn that when people are sad, they cry. It's more accurate to say that, when some people are sad, they cry. They may also show sadness by becoming quiet, or they may not externally show it at all. You can't tell everyone's emotional state from their actions if you're basing it off some limited *Ann & Barry* picture book.

We have no problem with the concept of biodiversity, do we? We accept that there is a variety of life on earth, from genes to flora and fauna to ecosystems. We also know that biodiversity is vital to sustain life. If there was no biodiversity, this would be a different planet, uninhabitable and hostile. Neurodiversity is a concept people seem to be a little bit slower to accept, however. 'What do you mean there are different types of brains?' Well there are.

Neurodiversity is a term that encompasses all brain types, from the 'typical' brain across a vast spectrum. Some people have brains that diverge from what is most common or typical, and those people – us wonderful and curious folk – can be described as neurodivergent. It's a term that represents a huge number of people living with many different diagnoses: ADHD, autism, dyslexia, dyspraxia and dyscalculia to name a few. I bet there is no one reading this who doesn't know at least one person with one of these labels. So, it's high time we began to accept that the world has been created by neurotypical people and does not meet the needs of the neurodivergent.

If we can accept this fully, then people may be able to go back a few steps and think more creatively about all the different ways the world can function. Can we rethink how work or school can be done? Can we make it more accessible to everyone? Because, let me assure you, having a neurodivergent person in your workplace is one foolproof way to ensure you are thinking outside the box, looking for patterns other people won't see, coming at problems from a different angle and considering the needs and wants of a whole new customer base you may have been missing.

It can often feel as though people are all on board for being inclusive and accepting until you actually ask for an accommodation from them. That's when the tone changes. As neurodivergent people, we get encouraged to drop the mask, to be our authentic selves. Then, when we do drop the mask, non-autistics don't like it and we get treated horribly because words are easy, but actions are harder.

Let's imagine that life is all about eating soup. As an autistic person, my brain – the tool I have been given to do life with – is a fork, but all the neurotypical people have been given a spoon. That's how I see it. Sometimes it can feel that the rhetoric around autism is around how I, the autistic person, can be supported in turning my fork into a spoon. Neurotypical people invite us to eat soup with them, they cheer us on because our fork is so unique and unusual, they tell us we are inspiring for continuing to try to eat alongside them. Some of them get annoyed when we spill soup all over ourselves or when it's taking us too long to finish and they're already done.

Why is it up to us to work impossibly hard, for impossibly long, to achieve an impossible task? It's not fair. I can't change my brain. I have a fork. It will always be a fork. Why can't it be up to you to put something on the menu that I can eat with a fork? That is the direction the world needs to move in. Yes, it will take more effort for you neurotypical people. Yes, it may take more time and be a little bit annoying. Yes, it may seem easier and simpler to hire someone, or teach someone, or befriend someone, who has the same utensil you have. But is that right? Is it fair?

We all have someone in our lives who's gone vegan and we still love and accept them as we fry their tofu don't we? I'm mixing metaphors but I think my point is clear.

Don't leave it to us to always be the ones trying to adapt. Meet us halfway at least.

All that said, I wouldn't swap my fork for a spoon if that were possible. There are things that are tough because I'm autistic, sure: unstructured socialising, managing friendships, coping with change, tolerating the sound of someone breathing … But, at the same time, the absolute best things about me are undoubtedly *because* I'm autistic.

After years of having a thirst for knowledge, coupled with my ability to memorise things, I am remarkably smart and know something about everything. I am loyal beyond belief, and sometimes to my detriment. If a company or institution treats me well and I have a first-name relationship with an employee, I will not switch company for any reason. Yes, I could get something cheaper elsewhere but cost isn't everything.

I have an innate sense of what is fair and right and I will die on any and every hill of injustice I see. I have a focus that is unmatched by any neurotypical person I know, and if you give me a deadline, I will never miss it. Punctuality is part of my being. I am thoughtful and remember tiny facts about what people like so I'm the best gift-giver. I spot patterns others don't see and it's very satisfying when people are impressed with the things I highlight that other people have missed.

Lastly, I'm delightfully unambiguous. I say what I mean and I mean what I say. If more people did that, the world would be a more peaceful and productive place.

Chandrika Narayanan-Mohan is an Irish-Indian writer, performer and cultural consultant, published by Dedalus Press, *Banshee*, *The Stinging Fly*, Poetry Ireland and others. She has been artist-in-residence for several science initiatives and is a Skein Press Play It Forward Fellow.

Rizz 'Em with the 'Tism

The title of this essay isn't going to age well. It is a phrase born from the wild reaches of neurodivergent Gen Z TikTok (via Instagram, where I, an ageing millennial, receive all my online content second-hand). Phrases like this have been shared by autistic people on social media lately, with 'rizz 'em with the 'tism' specifically alluding to quirkily seducing people with the charismatic magnetism of autistic flair. It's migrated from hashtags on screens into the real world, where I have witnessed someone walking down George's Street with the phrase emblazoned on a T-shirt. The idea that we're all out there being our actual unmasked selves, hooking up with cuties based on our ability to wax lyrical on special interests or shared delight, feels refreshing and affirming. What a time we're living in! I too want the phrase on a T-shirt.

The concept runs counter to a few things: firstly, the general assumption that autistic people are unable to have fulfilling and regular romantic and sexual connections with people, and secondly almost everything I've seen on *Love on the Spectrum*. A TV show about autistic adults looking for love, it features a cast of hopefuls including a man who proudly shows off his katana collection, a doe-eyed young woman who cuddles her toys and squeezes her eyes and mouth tightly shut when she chastely kisses her boyfriend, and two people faltering and lapsing into panicked silence while speed-dating. It makes for good TV: the high hopes and awkward scenes, the audience rooting for our earnest protagonists to achieve their dream and fall in love. Before the appearance of queer people a season later, it is also deeply heteronormative: there is much talk about finding The One, about marriage, kids, living the pre-*Frozen*-era Disney dream. Life appears to be hinging on this desire to couple up and settle, strongly endorsed by family members whose main fear is that they'll die and leave their autistic adult child to traverse the world alone. Now, I'm not here to shit on *Love on the Spectrum*, as these stories and relationships deserve airtime, and undoubtedly the experiences resonated with many viewers who felt affirmed and validated when seeing their stories on screen. For me personally, with the exception of one long-term couple whose story is quite lovely, the rest made for occasionally enlightening but fairly uncomfortable watching.

The thing is I wasn't watching for entertainment, I was watching for research. Despite being cheerfully solo, at age thirty-five I was interested in opening myself up to a certain type of love again after many years. I didn't feel a burning need to be in a relationship or in love, but I didn't want to run away from the possibility out of fear or ignorance. As a recently-diagnosed autistic person looking to potentially date again I wanted to gather information by watching this show, to see how other people like me manage romance, relationships, sex, how they communicate their needs and feelings, and how they are able to find partners who both accept and celebrate them for who they are, not in spite of it. Instead I was mostly faced with heartbreak, rejection, little to no examples of good communication, occasional moments of public humiliation, and DEFINITELY no sex.

I was disappointed. These were supposedly 'my people', but I struggled to find myself in any of those stories. I realised I wouldn't be 'autistic enough' to be on the show: I have no major special interests, no large room of collectibles, no extreme hyperfixation. Socialising is sometimes a challenge, but I am lucky that one of my best autistic skills is analysing and mapping social rules and networks so that I can navigate social situations mostly without incident. I have lived independently away from my family since the age of eighteen, and have had around twenty major relationships with generally decent people. However, my neurodivergence has played a large role in the collapse of these relationships and distressing experiences within them. I am aware the show's purpose was to choose the people who struggled the most with dating, but I was still disappointed to not see someone like me in the story. I suppose high-masking, burnt-out women just don't make for good reality TV.

And all of that is to say, it's a year later, and I am in love.

This is a sentence that might age as badly as the title of this essay, but it's true, and I am, and at the time of writing this, it's great. It wouldn't be my first rodeo: according to the Excel sheet I've put together of all my past relationships, by the age of thirty-six I have been in love sixteen times. When I say love, the grading system for love I am using in the spreadsheet is not nuanced: rating from one heart emoji to three heart emojis doesn't quite capture the breadth and depth of each love I have experienced. As a teenager, a quote from *Anna Karenina* caught my attention: 'If it is true that there are as many minds as there are heads, then there are as many kinds of love as there are hearts.' Which is all very well and good but difficult to convert into quantifiable criteria.

A part of being in love this time around does in fact involve spreadsheets. When discussing my neurodivergence, I often describe myself as 'the Excel sheet flavour of autism' because sometimes autism feels less like a spectrum and more like a Baskin-Robbins ice-cream counter. And for what feels like the first time in my life, I have found someone who is the same flavour as me. Within weeks of us dating, this person created a shared spreadsheet for us to negotiate everything from sensory needs to what movies we want to watch together. Communicating like this with someone who has a self-awareness and acceptance of their own neurodivergence has allowed me to be more open about mine. I am now realising how much I was struggling to fit into the mould of someone else's expectations in relationships, how obsessed I was with arbitrary criteria and other people's rules – and a lot of that was to do with a lack of understanding about neurodivergence.

This may sound like it's the first time I've been with someone neurodivergent, but that's not the case at all; if anything the opposite. After being diagnosed as autistic with ADHD (known also as AuDHD), and after reading books recommended to me by my psychiatrist, I found myself looking back though the list of past lovers and seeing a solid pattern of likely autism and ADHD emerge. But that didn't make things any easier for me, in fact during my most upsetting relationship it made it worse. I don't have the right to diagnose that person but all signs pointed to autism, just not the same flavour as mine: I can clearly see now where our logic systems clashed. I have since attempted to separate out what was actual bad behaviour and what were just autistic traits, and also identified times where I could have been much kinder and more understanding. And so after many years I find myself in love with someone with a similar brain to mine, and for once the sparks are flying in good ways.

Now, considering I criticised *Love on the Spectrum* for skirting conversations around sex and intimacy, it feels hypocritical to not address it myself. I am generally a very private person who doesn't discuss my relationships in public, but my therapist is currently on maternity leave so here we are, discussing autistic sex, immortalised on paper.

For many people sex and love don't have to be connected, but for me they have been since the beginning: I fell in love easily and prided myself on only sleeping with those people. At the time I had no idea that the term demisexual* existed, so didn't realise my lack of interest in one night stands was more to do with my wiring than my morals. I also felt more 'me' in open relationships, though as someone in their early twenties with no information about non-traditional relationship structures, I handled those terribly. Like demisexuality, I did not know the term polyamory existed, though if I had spent more time with the queer, kinky nerds on campus I would have learnt a lot more a lot faster! Speaking of kink, this was an area I had previously misunderstood and experienced with the wrong people in earlier years, but now it's a part of my life mostly due to the consideration of sensory needs, boundaries and conversation, queer expression, clear structures around power and clear communication needed in order to manage sex in an anxiety-free, safe and open manner.

---

* Demisexuality generally means that a person needs to have an emotional connection with someone before any sexual feelings can appear.

All these different aspects of my sexuality are twisted up together in me, previously tangled and confusing and often upsetting, but now finally woven into a tapestry of intimacy that makes sense. Turns out my period of asexuality was more about sensory issues, combined with an anxiety around intimacy and trust; my challenges with both poly relationships and serial monogamy finally made more sense as I understood how much ADHD and autism play into finding the balance of security and routine with novelty; and as a bisexual, my insecurity around relationships with women were less about being a 'bad gay' and more about those individual communication styles and needs that didn't align with mine, mostly because I had no idea how to even communicate my own needs and my own flavour of queerness. Autism weaves in and out through all these issues, and with more information about how my brain works, the anxieties and barriers have started to fall away as clear communication with the right kind of people has allowed for stronger bonds of trust, friendship, romance and intimacy. And yes, people plural, as I have finally come around to formalising my need for polyamory, with people who understand my brain, who are happy with what is on offer both in terms of the relationship structure and also what I bring to the relationship.

So yes, it's all falling into place, so what could possibly go wrong?

The ghosts of previous relationship failures hover at my ear during the good times, and with my mind repressing some of my memories, I struggle to remember how many times I've felt this way before, and am alarmed when realising I *have* felt this way before. Here is the familiar unlocking of the version of myself only ever witnessed by lovers; here are the old phrases of love and affection that tumble out across the tongue too easily; here are the plans and promises being laid like bricks, ones that were made before with people I am no longer with. Is this truly a moment of self-aware autistic love finally done right, or just another turn on the merry-go-round I can't remember being on before? Prior to my current relationships I don't remember who was the last person I said I love you to romantically, something which I would have said and heard on a daily basis at the time: it's a repressed memory I have been determined to recover, but to no avail. And also with more awareness comes more worries: will my ADHD kick in and will I suddenly get bored of a wonderful relationship? Is this really autistic unmasking or am I just mirroring a partner? Will my need for constant clarification and information be as off-putting as it's been described as before? Will my monologuing stop being cute and start being seen as self-indulgent and self-obsessed? Will my need for space and lack of touch be interpreted as cold and insensitive?

As I am sitting here listing out all these worries, my partner walks in and asks me, 'Are you in hyperfocus mode?', then offers to sit down next to me and watch cat videos on their phone so we can be together quietly.

A breath, a pause: the balloon of worry temporarily deflates.

It won't come as a surprise that my partner is a cat person. There are even memes about our kind of pairing, the golden retriever / black cat combo. And perhaps it's the combination of this person being both neurodivergent and good with cats that partly explains why they understand and love me for who I am. My cat-like behaviour has been a running joke amongst the people who know me, which

I now know is common with autistic people. I had always wondered why cats were allowed to exist comfortably as contradictory and contrary creatures – both affectionate and aloof, cuddly and angry, snoozy and chaotic, desperate for attention and then repulsed by it – and they were loved and accepted and I wasn't.

It may have taken a few decades, over ten years of therapy, various diagnoses, a lot of neurodivergent Instagram, and a heavy sprinkling of pure luck, but the time to live my best cat life has finally arrived. I can now spend as much time alone as I want and then be excited to spend time with my partners, without them finding that confusing. I can enjoy plenty of physical affection, but they don't feel rejected when I indicate that I don't want to be touched. In the past year there have been so many moments of neurodivergent joy shared with the people I love, whether it's quiet parallel play at home or giggling uncontrollably in an exhibition about dinosaurs. My intimate life feels powerful and comforting and free, brought about by an understanding of my own unique needs, and people who gently encourage me to figure out what they are and help me articulate them through different mediums. I am able to say 'I love you', able to practice saying and practice hearing it until it settles into my bones as truth. I am aware that this may change, but for once I trust that I will be informed properly if it does.

And with my partner's soft body resting next to mine as they scroll through their Instagram feed while I type on my laptop, it keeps boiling down to good moments like this. On my phone the chat with another partner is comfortably silent: every few days one of us throws a heart emoji into the chat to indicate *I am thinking of you / I love you*. Occasionally I will say the words themselves, so they have space to taste air, to settle into an easily articulated reassurance. With AuDHD communication as my compass, the issues that arose before are now less frightening and more unlikely, and I don't have to fight hard for the things that make me feel good and safe. I can co-exist intimately with another person, content in who I am and who we are together. For the first time I don't feel like I am too much or not enough: I simply am. And in these moments I can, for a few minutes at least, stop dissecting what it is to be deeply and autistically in love and instead just savour the fact that I am.

Emil E. Osiński is a male, 25-year-old Polish writer who has lived in Ireland for seventeen years. Emil specialises in poetry, plays and personal essays, but has tried his hand at novel and short-story writing as well as screenwriting. He uses writing as a way to raise awareness of topics such as mental health in men and familial abuse.

I'm So Burnt Out I Can Smell the Smoke

Recently I suffered a severe autistic burnout, which is best described as chronic exhaustion, loss of skills and very low tolerance to stimuli. I didn't have the time to take care of it properly, and it resulted in me completely breaking down at work. I came to work in the morning feeling panicky and exhausted. It was as though there was a fog around my head, clouding my vision, muting the voices of other people, but the noise of the machines and children crying was ever so loud. I was working the floor, washing tables, picking up trays and putting them and the dishes into the dishwasher. It was already busy, and I had no energy to be as quick as I usually was. Then the first rush of the day happened, people started pouring in as though we had a special event going on, and I was asked to help behind the counter. I knew I couldn't do it, but didn't have much of a choice.

I was put on the coffee shots, but I was way too slow. My brain in some way knew what to do, but I felt like I was moving in tar, so I was more in the way than I was being helpful. My manager noticed that I was slowing everything down and angrily told me to go on the milk instead. That did it for me. I freaked out and started crying in front of all those customers. Unable to work or leave, I was just frozen in place.

My manager thought I was just scared by the rush, but when she realised it wasn't the case she guided me into the kitchen, so I could calm down. She asked what happened, but I just talked about some recent events in my life, since I couldn't tell her that I was overwhelmed; that I didn't know working again after three years and in such a place would make my shutdowns so much worse. I was too scared that if I told her, she would be angry at me and potentially ask me to resign, because at the interview I swore I was well able for this type of job. We sat in the office as she tried to get someone to cover my shift. Unfortunately no one was available, and I still had about seven or so hours to go.

The majority of people step into a made-up version of themselves when going to a job interview. You have to appear confident, intelligent, knowledgeable, easy-going, and all the best things the employer might be looking for. It's not much different for autistic people, except there's a lot more hiding involved. I've been looking for work on and off for the past two years. Anytime I was given an interview and mentioned it to any non-autistic person I knew, they always told me the same things: 'You have to keep eye contact' … 'Don't play with your hands'… 'If you're not confident, just pretend'… 'Don't mention *this* or *that* interest'. I never gave it much thought. I grew up undiagnosed, I needed to fit in, so I got used to doing what I was told. The interviews almost never led anywhere anyway, and when they did, it was some cleaning jobs where the biggest stress was having to suddenly leave the apartment we were cleaning and clean a different apartment before finishing a previous one, because of last-minute bookings. It wasn't until I was employed at a coffee shop that I started thinking more about how stupid this game of pretence is, and for the first time ever I wondered whether I could keep pretending past the interview.

The place I currently work at is not some small, side-street café that barely anyone visits and the biggest rush consists of ten people. It's one of the bigger chains, where they push towards not only quality service, but also very quick service. We have rushes that can last for hours with people ordering cakes, pastries, sandwiches to be toasted, iced drinks, coffees, not too hot, extra hot, not too much syrup, whip, not too much whip, cream, no cream, soya milk, coconut, oat, skimmed, less froth, more froth – everyone has their preference. Owing to our location, families, the elderly and caregivers of disabled people are our most frequent customers.

During the interview I did what I was told: kept eye contact, pretended to be confident, talked about how much I would love to work with people, how well I work in a team, exaggerated my skills, and I got the job. But now what? I am autistic. This is a part of me that I cannot erase. And there are things you cannot mask, such as autistic burnouts, getting easily overwhelmed and because of it, often going nonverbal, and inability (in my case) to remember anything that's told as a list, inability to read tone or use the correct tone.

In places like this, stimming is completely out of the question as it makes me appear nervous. Stimming is something that autistic people do to manage emotions or self-regulate, such as repetitive body movements or movements of objects, or repetition of words or sounds. It's different for everyone; I personally play with my hands or any strings I can find. All through my life stimming had been perceived as nervousness, from my mother saying 'If I ever find out down the line that there's something you're not telling me, it'll break my heart' because she thought my stimming was nervousness, and thus I must be hiding something from her, to my career-guidance teacher ending our conversation prematurely because I was 'clearly too nervous', or my manager telling me 'no need to stress' when I just needed to stim. Listing out the order to the customer before I ask them to pay is frowned upon, as it makes it seem like I wasn't listening. I was, I do this because it helps me make sure there are no misunderstandings. Eye contact is mandatory in order to make the customer feel welcome. I struggle with eye contact, and no matter how hard I try, I never find the right balance. Either I stare into the person's eyes or keep darting around their face, neither of which are good. Noise is everywhere because of families, people having conversations, blenders, coffee machines, but I can't wear earplugs to drown it out. I have to be alert, listen out for new orders. It's difficult when my ears hurt, and I'm so overwhelmed I want to cry.

An environment like this, paired with the constant masking, has led to more severe autistic burnouts than I have ever experienced before, while I try to balance it with my numerous hobbies that I do after work. All the things I have learnt about myself and my autistic identity since I got diagnosed, above all how to take care of myself, are impossible to implement. I cannot just withdraw to a quiet place, put music on and stim during rush hour, or when the day is very busy. In my previous jobs I was able to listen to my music and work alone, as we split the tasks and sections. The only time I had to mask was during lunch, unless I chose to go somewhere else to eat.

Since the meltdown, I've started to wake up with anxiety on the days I work, and it never passes until I've worked for at least an hour. This was the first time something like this happened at work, but I know very well that unless I figure out the right balance and new techniques for managing autistic burnouts, this will happen again. It happened a couple of times when I was still in school, but back then I was just sent to the councillor's office. Now I could end up being asked to resign as it's obvious I'm 'not the right fit for this kind of job'. The patience of non-autistic people runs out so quickly when you need more accommodations than an average person, especially when you're an adult asking for accommodations. It's as though non-autistic people believe that the older we get, the 'less autistic' we become. It may seem that way when we're taught to mask from a very early age, but the autism doesn't just disappear.

I want to prove to myself that I can do this, that my autistic identity is in no way a burden or something standing in the way of my success – instead it's something to embrace and celebrate. All my life I pushed that 'me' down and punished him for things he never deserved to be punished for, just because everyone around me did it to me. The only question is, how do I make accommodations for myself that work both at home and at work? As my routine got interrupted by a different work schedule every week, I created a new one for days that I work. I come in at least half an hour early so I can make myself coffee, sit down in peace, and drink it before I switch to work mode. It's not much compared to my routine on my days off, but it does involve having coffee in peace, so that helps.

This gives me some hope that maybe there are small things I can do for myself that will prevent my autistic burnouts from reaching a point like this again. Being autistic shouldn't stop me from being able to function in society. I want to learn how to reach out for help as well. Doing everything alone is only going to make this worse in the long run. I'm lucky to have a boss who tries her best to understand my struggles, and if I need it, she does give me a day off. I am autistic, I can't change this, but with the right people in my life, and a lot of patience and understanding from myself towards myself, I will be able to do just fine and never again have to hide this part of me.

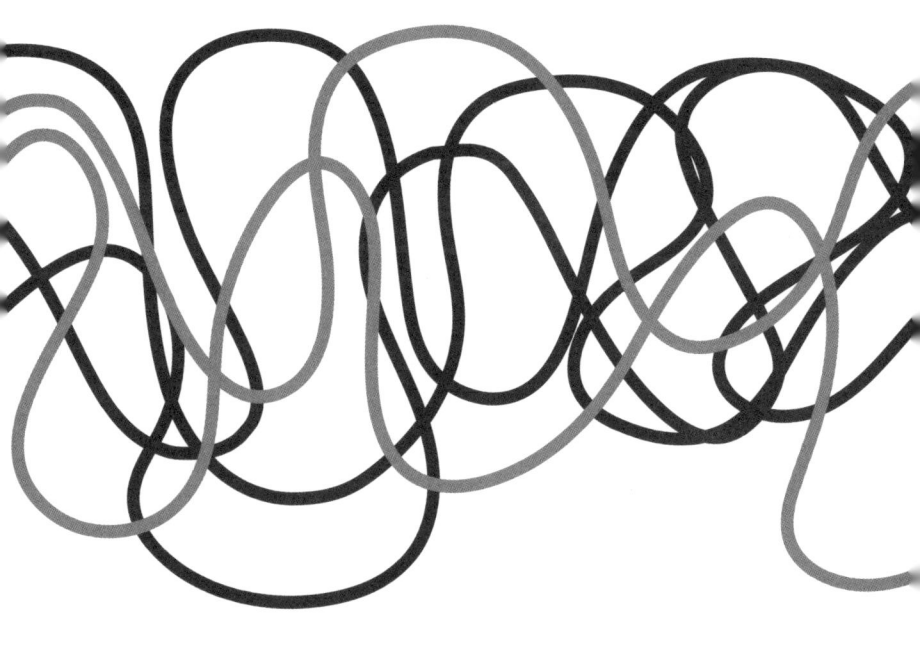

Stuart Neilson is an autistic statistician and writer. He combines his writing with images describing his experience of public spaces, most often in his home city of Cork.

Sharing Spaces

Our public places are full of rich sensory experiences. Sensory aspects are important to the ambience of places, such as the noisy 'buzz' of a popular café, and the character of products, such as the 'new car' smell. However, like many autistic people, I find that too much sensory input tires me out and limits my ability to get things done.

My biggest triggers are unpredictable sounds, flashing displays that constantly snag my attention, inappropriate food odours (such as strawberry-scented disinfectant) and skin contact. A lack of decent signs and directions – and unexpected changes – are also difficult for me. This could be something as simple as not recognising where to queue or order in a café, or an extra checkout opening in the supermarket, leaving me lost and dithering while everyone else seems to know what they are doing. The general sense of anxiety raised by sensory overload distracts my attention from whatever I am doing, and adds effort to activities in public places. When these activities involve other people, I am distracted from fully concentrating on them and from fully engaging with conversation.

Alexithymia – literally 'not having words for feelings' – means that I feel the full intensity of emotions and bodily senses, but I cannot quickly tell what they are. Just over half of autistic people are also alexithymic. We cannot always tell emotions apart, or tell senses apart, and cannot always distinguish between emotions and senses. A full bladder can feel to me like anxiety or being too hot. Sometimes I don't recognise an emotion or sensation until I have had a day or more to process the feelings.

Before I became aware of being autistic, I attributed the feelings of sensory load to social friction, and it caused me a great deal of stress and anxiety because I constantly felt people were watching and judging me. I was diagnosed fifteen years ago while being treated for depression and anxiety, at the age of forty-five. Diagnosis made a tremendous difference to me, because I was suddenly connected to a global community of autistic people and their experiences, and to a label that explained my own experiences. My feelings of exclusion, otherness and not belonging in social environments are largely a consequence of the difficulties I have with sensory overload and anxiety, and not my fault. The label has been very positive in directing me towards resources describing how to cope better in difficult environments, and also to the idea that environments could be different, could be more welcoming. The label also helps shift the burden away from my failure to manage in demanding sensory environments and towards the people who choose to make places that are noisy, visually jarring and full of intense odours.

Sensory sensitivity never goes away, but I have found some ways to reduce the anxiety it causes me. I wear noise-cancelling headphones on the bus or train, where I feel safe away from traffic, but more often I wear a thick woollen hat to muffle the most intrusive noises. I always wear long sleeves and a thick coat if the weather is not too hot to avoid skin contact, wet things, breezes and being jostled in crowds. I have identified places where I feel calm, and times of day when those places are most calm. I try to identify refuge places – the library, bookshops and parks – beyond where I need to go for my essential daily activities, and quieter routes connecting them. This means I have a safe place to spend a little time if I arrive early for an appointment, and places to walk to when I want more exercise.

Occasionally I hide my difficulty processing words by holding a hand behind my ear, as if I have not heard what someone said, when in reality I heard the sounds of the words quite clearly, but they make no sense until later. Most people slow down and say what they meant again using different words instead of just repeating it. Between the extra time this allows me to process what they said first and the alternative words, I usually have time to understand what they meant. Disclosure can be really helpful, whether that is by directly identifying myself as autistic (perhaps on hospital visits where I need to be warned before anyone touches me, and in a small number of friendly shops I use), or by displaying some kind of symbol. I have used the AsIAm ID Card in medical visits, and I keep it in my wallet just in case it helps if I become distressed and hospital staff misinterpret a meltdown as overreaction. I wear a sunflower lanyard when travelling, with a JAM (Just a Minute) card reading *Please be patient, I am autistic*. It has been extremely helpful in many airports to smooth interactions with check-in and security staff.

Avoiding discomfort might seem like an effective way to control the anxiety caused by public places. Going somewhere quieter, taking calmer (usually longer) routes, or just staying at home all seem like effective solutions. They are also a form of self-exclusion and lead to a loss of opportunity for education, work, leisure or desirable social interaction. There is a trade-off between the discomfort of using public places and the rewards of doing so. Getting out more, anywhere, is also vital to getting enough physical activity for lifelong physical and mental well-being, especially as I have grown older. Trying to fit in, or trying to blend into the background, also seem like useful ways to minimise social discomfort. If nobody notices me, or nobody notices I am autistic, surely it will be more comfortable? This is true up to a point, but masking takes a lot of energy to do well, and can be exhausting. I know from my alexithymia and my own past mental health crises that I do not recognise that I am exhausted until I am already burned out.

As I have got older and experienced physical illness, I have become much more aware of difficulties with proprioception and my inability to correctly judge the distances between my body and other people or obstacles. Walking down a busy street has always been hard, trying to avoid accidentally walking into other people in motion. Becoming less balanced creates an additional need to have secure footing, space to balance, and surfaces that are comfortable and clean enough to touch for support. I have become more aware of and reliant on inclusive and accessible public places.

Good design can alleviate many of the daily challenges autistic people experience. Places with a choice of acoustics, calm escape spaces, clear guidance and easy interaction with staff make the difference between being included and being excluded from opportunities. This is especially important in healthcare settings. For example, it is often difficult for me to make, reschedule or confirm a healthcare appointment because I do not like making (and especially dislike answering) telephone calls. The waiting rooms tend to be over-bright and sometimes have no seats away from daytime TV or a noisy vending machine. It takes effort to get timely treatment, to attend health screening programmes and to understand health advice. My difficulty processing and responding to spoken words gets worse under pressure, so I sometimes don't understand or ask staff to clarify important verbal communications under these stressful conditions.

The spatial design of a place influences the emotions we feel in that place and the social interactions that are possible within it. Good design can enable, encourage or enforce inclusive practices. A place can encourage accessibility when it directs people to use space with care for others, for instance by having a range of spaces that are quieter and noisier by design, allowing people to gravitate to their chosen comfort level. Some places enforce accessibility with marked queuing points, social-distance indicators and signposted quiet areas. In contrast, some smaller shops and cafés do not clearly signpost how to queue or order. I cannot cope with the free-for-all crowding and error messages of self-service digital payment – but I hope both staffed and self-checkout options will remain for people who need them.

The sensory environments in cafés, shops, workplaces and hospitals are choices, and profoundly influence accessibility and inclusion for people with invisible disabilities. Accessible design that is fully inclusive is better for everyone. Nothing that is good for autistic people is bad for people who are not autistic, and in many cases is preferable to everyone.

Most people attribute the treatment I have had for depression, my long periods of unemployment and my limited social interactions directly to being autistic. We need to completely overturn these views. Lower expectations, limited employment opportunities, difficulty accessing healthcare, lower levels of satisfaction and reduced social engagement are barriers imposed on us by others. Autistic people experience lifelong marginalisation, exclusion and limited opportunities because society treats us differently. There is also evidence that autistic people have shorter lifespans than non-autistic people.

If only it was more widely understood that the many limitations autistic people experience are the consequence of stigma and exclusion – and not the natural or inevitable outcomes of being autistic.

Further Information:
Magda Mostafa's ASPECTSS design framework: autism.archi/aspectss

Dublin City University's *Autism-Friendly University Design Guide*: dcu.ie/commsteam/news/2021/jun/dcu-launches-first-ever-autism-friendly-university-design-guide

AsIAm Ireland: asiam.ie/what-we-do/training-accreditation

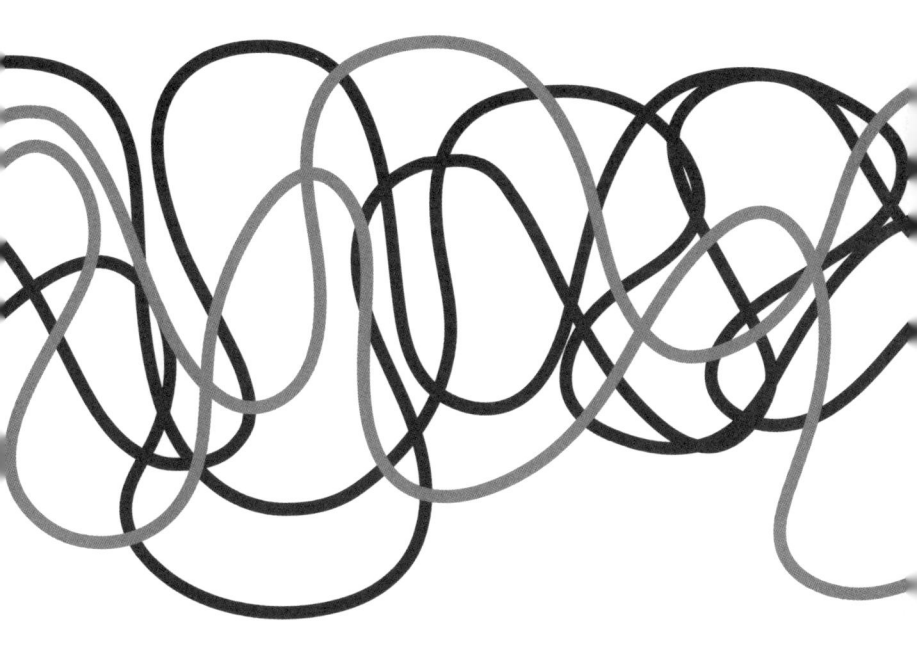

Caoimhe O'Gorman is a nineteen-year-old college student studying pharmaceutical science. Diagnosed with autism in 2022, Caoimhe now wants to share her experience to help others just starting their diagnosis journey.

A Tale of Two Lockdowns

The lockdown was a strange time for all of us. It's something that shook the foundations of our society, forcing us to undergo a period of readjustment no one knew how to navigate. Its aftershocks resulted in a trauma we haven't even begun to unpack. But in the midst of all that chaos, the lockdown saved me.

You read that correctly, a lockdown saved my life.

That time spent inside, alone with no outside noise, was transformative. That isn't to say the lockdown wasn't a stressful and scary time, but I think I was one of the lucky ones. My social life largely stayed the same. I hadn't gone out much before the pandemic on account of my sensitivity to crowds, bright lights and loud noises. I also mainly talked to my friends over the internet, so I wasn't suddenly cut off from them either. Other than the anxiety around my family and my health and keeping each other safe, I didn't experience many growing pains adjusting to Covid life.

At the time I was fourteen years old and just starting my third year in secondary school. I hadn't yet been diagnosed and couldn't begin to believe I was autistic. I was everything the stereotype of autism said couldn't possibly be autism. I was independent and excelled academically. I didn't have a natural affinity for maths. Most importantly I was able to cage the meltdowns away until I got home and could release everything in private.

During a meltdown it becomes mechanically difficult to talk. Often all I can do is cry for hours at a time, just to try and release the energy trapped inside me. I tend to just pick a thing and stare at it, I grit my teeth until they hurt and appear like a wounded animal to all those around me. Except my wounds aren't physical, they are mental and wholly difficult to identify and communicate to others. Afterwards, I feel sluggish and numb, I find it difficult to gauge if I'm hungry, thirsty, or tired and need to be prompted to resolve any of these feelings.

My friends and my teachers never saw me melt down, something I'd purposely hidden because I was ashamed. I didn't know they were autistic meltdowns for a long time and instead thought I was just too sensitive. I assumed I was quiet, introverted and socially awkward. But then the unexplained, crushing anxiety came.

At times it felt like a giant was standing on my chest. The anxiety began to impede my ability to function and I was growing unhappier by the day. Before Covid the gaps in my school attendance were growing longer; I was going into school and having to be sent home only a half an hour into the day because I was physically sick from the stress. I was still performing academically so allowances were made and still I didn't want to acknowledge it was a problem, even when my family tried to tell me otherwise. Probably because I didn't want to admit that I wasn't completely 'normal'. So, I suppressed my burnout, refusing to acknowledge it, until soon enough it became this looming 'thing' I couldn't escape. I'd spent most of my life up to that point unconsciously masking my autistic qualities that society found undesirable, and it'd grown exhausting. I felt ashamed. I felt like a land mine that had arrived in the post without a diffusion manual. I believed I would blow up everyone I loved. The lockdown allowed me to finally break down in safety. I shed the protective coating I'd encased myself in for years and started anew, rebuilding from the ground up.

For the first time in my life, with no one except my family around, who I knew wouldn't judge me, I could stop trying to act 'normal', I could just be. I could finally just be me.

I've never liked people standing so close to me. I experienced it as an invasion of my personal space and as a physical threat and a major discomfort. Now because of the lockdown we were all mandated to a two-metre social-distance bubble. Covid gave me a justifiable reason for wanting to keep my distance. Previously my peers would throw their arms around each other at the drop of a hat, but I'd always shied away from such casual physical touch. In the lockdown the closest I got to touching was an elbow bump and the odd hug from those in my family who always knew how to properly touch me, even from a young age. I don't think we discussed, we just seemed to fall into it after a bit of trial and error. It was some unspoken rule that I initiate physical contact, or my family ask if I want a hug, for example. In addition to this we began to ask each other if we wanted a firm or gentle hold, which helped enormously.

On the whole, online schooling was a breeze; I didn't have to wear the scratchy uniform that made my skin itch or ask an adult for permission to leave the classroom, sometimes to use the bathroom but other times just to have a break from the constant activity. As it seemed no matter what excuse I gave, none were satisfactory or at the right time. I wasn't forced to abide by some arbitrary timetable telling me when I could eat. I didn't have to deal with rowdy classmates who didn't want to be in school. I didn't have to manicure myself to meet neurotypical fashion expectations. I didn't have to be concerned about my facial expressions (or lack thereof) being misconstrued. Social distancing made shopping easier because I wasn't as jumpy around people clogging up the aisles, because there were just fewer people. Plus, there was less dawdling inside the shops, it was in and out as quickly as possible, treating it like a mission instead of recreation. As neurotypicals seemed to keel over at each new restriction, I was largely unbothered and even began to experience increased freedom and ease.

All around me people on social media and on television were lamenting their troubles, honestly describing how the lockdown was affecting their mental health. But I felt fine. Out of seemingly everyone in the world, I was OK, and I began to wonder why.

After plenty of research everything seemed to point to autism, so with the support of my family I went for an assessment and as we emerged from the pandemic, my assessment confirmed what I already knew to be true, I was autistic. This diagnosis simultaneously changed everything and yet changed nothing. Being armed with an explanation as to why I am the way I am was comforting and helped me learn how to better take care of myself. But it didn't change how other people treated me. Life just carried on. As lockdown restrictions were gradually lifted, I had to readjust. In fact, it wasn't until things began to go back to 'normal' that I began to experience trauma. I was terrified of having to go back to my life before Covid because it was only through the lockdowns that I realised how truly unhappy I was. Partly because I was convinced that what I was going through wasn't a big deal and that I could get through it. But that stopped once I went an entire week without having a meltdown, without getting sick from the stress, and getting more than six hours of sleep a night.

I don't claim to represent all autistic voices, but my lockdown experience was the closest I've ever felt to living in a world built with me in mind. I could live peacefully without constant obstacles. I understand that my experience is not true for neurotypicals; largely they seemed to feel the exact opposite to me, like their world order was ending. At every perceived narrowing of social possibilities and lack of socialising, they panicked. The majority felt unsettled and adrift, unable to navigate the current.

They felt they were sinking under the pressure of the new rules of a society they hadn't opted into.

But I could move through our locked-down world with ease, without my usual triggers. I guess this is how neurotypicals feel every day. I didn't feel out of place or that I stuck out like a sore thumb, I was following the same rules as everybody else, except they were like second nature to me. The rules just made sense to me; I couldn't understand why neurotypicals had such a huge problem following the rules because they were all so logical. Why would we touch all the time, or stand so close together, or congregate in big groups? Science was telling us we needed to follow these rules to keep each other safe. Up until that moment, knowing their place in the world and feeling secure in that thought was a privilege neurotypicals didn't realise they possessed.

This leads me to believe that neurotypicals understanding our plight is not as impossible a proposition as we may think. Because they already have experienced our discomfort, a small portion of it anyway, through the lockdown, where for the first time neurotypicals had to live in a world at odds with what they felt was normal or natural.

What I realised through all this is that the panic neurotypicals felt during the lockdown is what it feels like for us every day to walk around in their world. Through the pandemic they have unintentionally walked a mile, or several, in our shoes. We all need to remember what it was like for all of us during those weird years. Neurotypicals need to remember the levels of distress they felt so they can better empathise with us. And autistic people need to hold onto how we felt during the lockdown, how much easier it was without the standard triggers of everyday life. We can carve out our place in the world now, using life during the lockdown as a blueprint. For me that took the form of eventually deciding to study for my Leaving Cert from home and I'm happy to say meltdowns have become more an irregularity rather than routine. Before the lockdown and before my diagnosis I was terrified of what I was feeling, terrified the meltdowns would never end. But because of the lockdown I gained tools that allow me to see the overwhelm coming. I learnt to take steps that mitigate it before it upgrades to a fully-fledged meltdown. And finally how to care for myself, how to pick up the pieces after the storm rolls through and carry on with my life. This is a continued effort I must make, to organise my life in a way that works for me and not how society dictates I should live. It involves taking things slowly, doing things that may seem strange to others, no matter how different.

As a society, we still have a lot of work to do, choosing to exercise compassion every day, not jumping to judgement based on how someone may seem on the outside. We all need to remember that shared feeling of community and care we had for each other during the lockdown, despite our differences. Because if we can hold onto that, then the future is brighter if only for the fact that I know we're in it together.

Adam Harris is an autistic advocate and the founder–CEO of AsIAm, Ireland's autism charity. A Social Entrepreneurs Ireland awardee, Adam is a member of the Irish Human Rights and Equality Commission and the Executive Committee of Autism Europe.

My Path to Advocacy

My mum always says that I never do anything until I am ready and then I do it very quickly. That in fact started at birth: I was twenty days overdue and born in twenty-five minutes! From the moment I was born, I had a huge attachment to my mum in particular, and she couldn't put me out of her arms for two minutes without me seeking her out or becoming distressed. This meant I didn't sleep in my own bed, or for more than a few hours a night, until I was seven years old.

From when I was really young, I developed passionate interests which I could focus on intensely and learn everything about. This included time-bound interests in TV shows or children's series through to a lifelong love of facts, current affairs and history. I was around five years old when I first came across a book on Tutankhamun and Ancient Egypt and this lit a fire in me in terms of a love of history that has remained with me ever since. Despite this, the world felt a very overwhelming place. It was too noisy, too busy, too smelly and too demanding. Other children didn't seem to share my interests. Going new places or dealing with the day-to-day stressors of pre-school, family occasions or changes in plan could be very distressing. I stimmed a lot and would seek out quiet corners away from others in pre-school, but couldn't explain why I needed to do this. I couldn't yet articulate my differences, so my parents also had to figure out new ways to support me. At the time, this was far from easy – accessing an autism diagnosis was not straightforward (as is still too often the case today) and often other adults or people in the community could be quick to label me as 'bold' or 'difficult'. When I was diagnosed, my parents found that others in our community didn't necessarily know what it meant to be autistic or how best to support and include me.

Growing up in the late 1990s and early 2000s, my family always tried to speak to me about autism in positive terms. I am often asked, 'Should I or should I not tell my child that they are autistic?' This comes in the context of people wanting to understand *when* I had learnt about my diagnosis and the positives, or otherwise, that this knowledge brought me. I always had to be honest with people and say that knowledge of my autistic identity forms part of some of my earliest memories. Of course, we didn't use the same words or terminology that we would today, and the societal implications of that identity were certainly very different, but nonetheless my parents always spoke openly to me. I can remember my mum saying things to me like, 'You know the way you know all the flags of the world, but you don't like going to busy places? Well that is called autism.' I remember my family being always willing to challenge those who would stare if I became distressed in public places and insist that I had as many opportunities to participate in my own local community as possible.

You cannot separate your experiences and sense of identity from the prevailing attitudes and values of the society in which you grow up. If my own family's attitudes to autism were positive, the narrative and mood music surrounding autism were anything but.

When I look back through old files in my house I find newspaper clippings, leaflets promoting talks and other literature which promote everything from so-called 'cures' and 'treatments' to an overtly negative, medicalised view of what it meant to be autistic. Given that this was the information available to families, it almost goes without saying that awareness (let alone understanding or acceptance) was far from universal in the society at large. Whether it was sitting next to me in pre-school or principals responding to my parents' queries about enrolment, people were quite direct in their outlook on my support needs or right to participate. Some parents of children in playschool and other activities were reluctant for their child to interact with me. Activity-providers, and even public services such as schools, had no hesitation in saying they didn't provide for children 'like that'. Even as the number of people accessing assessment increased, so too did the misconceptions, rumours and snake oil surrounding the community. As the conversation grew, it was a conversation *about* autistic people and doing things *to* autistic people, with the voices *of* autistic people painfully absent.

It was against this backdrop that I started my education in a special school, far from my community in the millennium year, without access to the curriculum or subjects that I was interested in and would have excelled at – from my love of flags and capital cities to my passion for all things historical. While I had many positive experiences in the special school, it was a welcome moment when I was around seven years old and my mum first said to me, 'Do you think you could ever go into a local national school with the support of an SNA?'

I read *The Curious Incident of the Dog in the Night-Time* when I was around ten years old. In my innocence I saw my differences as wholly a thing with which I should have no fear or shame in being associated. When I was a little bit older, however, I began to see the very real implications of being autistic in Irish society. Like any young person or teenager, I wanted to feel and be the same as everyone else. Activities such as socialising, accessing resources in school or asking for reasonable accommodations, which felt easy and achievable in my early years in primary school, suddenly began to seem very difficult and draining as I progressed towards secondary school. I have often described the gap that opened up as being reminiscent of a scene in the airport, with others cruising along on the travelator and me sprinting next to it trying to keep up. On the one hand, this was challenging as I needed to learn to embrace my differences and be comfortable with going my own way. On the other, though, it was clear that society encouraged sameness and conformity, and had different expectations of me because of my neurotype. Whether it was people's well-intentioned desire to protect me rather than give opportunities for independence or the stereotypical view of autism that others in the community could often have, there was often an assumption that I couldn't do things; not based on identified support needs, but due to the word 'autism' alone.

This stigma surrounds the word. From around the age of eleven I hated anyone knowing I was autistic and would refuse to engage in programmes or supports that were made available to me; sometimes because of fear of association and other times because the support was not designed in an empowering or affirming way. When I started secondary school, and parted with many of my peers from sixth class, I was determined that no one in secondary school would know about my diagnosis and that I would do everything for myself. This, of course, was a recipe for disaster. On the one hand, demands on me were growing and, on the other, my self-esteem and willingness to access reasonable accommodations were diminishing. Around this time I had two seminal conversations which would greatly help me on my advocacy journey, in very different ways. One was with an amazing teacher in school who reminded me that part of achieving the independence I was seeking was to embrace my differences and be willing to accept the accommodations I would need to make it a reality. The other was with a person in the community who asked me in a queue in a shop would I not be sitting my Junior Cert – the implication being because I was autistic. In a sense, as things improved for me the following year, these were the two key messages in the back of my mind – one that I should be proud and open about who I am and the second that this was only possible by also educating others.

It was during my transition year that I first had the idea to establish a blog to share my experiences with others and to try and break down the sense of isolation I had so keenly felt in the previous years. I was around sixteen when I called a meeting in the International Bar in Dublin and the seeds were planted for what became AsIAm, Ireland's Autism Charity.

In my first piece, which I wrote on a blog that I'd called AspergersAdvice.org, I said, 'I know anyone who has tried to communicate with me as they were speaking to me as E.T. does so with the best of intentions.' This captured both my personal sense of shame and stigma, and the early stage Ireland was at in moving from a medicalised view of autism towards truly neuro-affirmative society. This blog was shared widely on social media and led me to giving a host of print, radio and television interviews in the summer of 2012, culminating in an appearance on *The Late Late Show* that November.

Whereas today I wouldn't think twice about owning my autistic identity, it is fair to say that from the time I was a pre-teen through to the day I wrote the article, I hated other people knowing that I was autistic. There was a real sense of almost contradictory isolation. On the one hand, a sense that you were the only young person experiencing the whirlwind that is growing up as an autistic person in Ireland; and, on the other, a recognition that you were a member of a secret society, in which you knew other autistic people in your community but it wasn't discussed and a pervasive stigma remained. Even after I wrote the piece, I was very cautious around my own peers, particularly those with whom I had developed hard-won friendships, and those I interacted with who knew that I was autistic. I would abruptly change the conversation if asked about it in my local community and even as I began to blog and give daytime television interviews, I did it secure in the knowledge that I was largely speaking to adult strangers and that not too many sixteen- or seventeen-year-olds were paying attention to those kinds of media channels.

It was only when I appeared on *The Late Late Show* that most of my own friends found out about my diagnosis for the first time! Yes, they knew I was different and yes, they knew I accessed some supports in secondary school, and yet I feared embracing that difference fully or putting a name to it for fear of being judged or treated differently.

Moving beyond stigma is a process not a moment, and for many years I remained reluctant to engage with supports including when I started university, dropping out shortly afterwards.

Since then, it has been an incredible privilege to get to know so many autistic people and families across the country, to see our proud community find its voice, and the emergence of an extraordinary momentum towards building a more inclusive society in Ireland. As I began to travel around the country, meeting other autistic people and families, I was constantly surprised by just how similar the experiences and feelings of other autistic people were to my own. It was only through the work I was doing with AsIAm that I felt the sense of a lid being lifted and the opportunity to correct the dominant narrative around autism, which seemed often detached or at least an incomplete telling of the lived experiences of our community.

It is worth pausing to reflect on how much society has changed since my school and college years. There have never been higher levels of public awareness of autism, with over 80 per cent of those surveyed in a recent AsIAm poll confirming they were aware of the term. Once seen as something unusual or relatively rare, one in twenty-seven children in our school system now has an autism diagnosis and we see more and more adults access diagnosis through private channels each year. There is huge work to be done to remove the often invisible barriers that exist for many of us. There is also a momentum across Irish society with countless schools, workplaces and even towns and cities seeking to take steps to give autistic people the same chance. Perhaps the greatest shift of all has been the rise of autistic voices in Ireland. Self-advocacy has greatly expanded the public's knowledge of and empathy towards our experiences – indeed, in the same poll those who reported being aware of an autistic person in their own life were much more likely to have positive viewpoints of autistic people. As we know from other areas of social change, it is not ultimately facts or statistics that lead to great leaps forward but a recognition by the general public that the experiences of autistic people are not just the subject of academic literature, but the day-to-day lives of their family, neighbours, colleagues and friends. A positive indicator that this shift will further grow in the years ahead is that over 50 per cent of those represented in our recent poll now reported knowing a person with a diagnosis of autism, of which almost half pointed to an immediate or extended family member.

This is the fruits of trailblazing autistic advocates, families and allies who have campaigned, litigated, trained and organised to break down barriers and create the environment in which change is truly possible. The progress did not come just in the last twenty years, building from a very low base, but rather from the labours of those who fought to end some of the most horrific practices of institutionalisation globally, going back to the foundations of the State. I am often asked by older people, 'Why did I not hear about this when I was in school?' with the sad, truthful answer being that Ireland was a society that hid difference, stigmatised disability and segregated all forms of diversity. When we consider that context, it is hard to understand that we are living in the same country today. That said, we most certainly cannot fall into the fallacy of clicking stop or allowing an idea to take root that we have an inclusive society today.

When the time for change comes, and a community builds, the pace it can gather is unfathomable. It has been nothing short of incredible to watch the evolution of the autism community over the past decade. From language and symbols, to shifting priorities and the diversity of voices, our community today is unrecognisable and so much stronger than it was in the year in which AsIAm was founded. This shift has not only had an internal effect in our community but has begun to reflect in our society, too slowly given the scale of the challenges that persist and yet far faster than any of us could truly have believed possible. AsIAm has grown from being an information website, run from my bedroom, to a national, autistic-led organisation with a large national footprint – providing neuro-affirmative support directly to autistic people and helping to build a more accessible society for us all to enjoy. The autism community generally has grown in every direction with each year seeing powerful new voices, groups, grassroots campaigns and initiatives that are yielding results on the ground. The shift away from a pathologised, medicalised view of autism is slowly being reflected in national policy, public services and in the world of work. Yet, there is a sense that we are only getting warmed up. Today we celebrate the breaking down of each individual barrier, big and small, but we will know we have succeeded when the expectation and experience of full equality is felt by every autistic person, in every aspect of Irish life.

AsIAm's 2024 Same Chance Report shows this is still a long way off. Whether it is accessing a school place, accessing education while in school, securing employment, enjoying a high quality of life or having a sense of safety, value and inclusion in the community, pervasive barriers still exist. It is appropriate that as advocates we continue to point out that awareness has been achieved. Understanding and acceptance must now urgently follow.

If there was one insight I could offer in the journey we must support Irish society to go on in the coming decade, it is the need to reassess the root causes of the attitudinal barriers our community faces. Each year in the AsIAm public poll 'Attitudes to Autism' we have asked a series of questions on knowledge of autism such as 'Have you heard of autism?' 'Would you be friends with us?' 'Would you hire us?' 'Do you think the government and society needs to do more to support us?' Year on year, the public strongly agreed with us. This year, the poll didn't ask people about autism. At least, not to begin with. We started by asking about day-to-day interactions in which our community has highlighted discrimination, such as 'Do you think a person should go to the cinema or theatre if they can't sit still or be quiet?', 'Do you think a child should be punished for becoming distressed in school?', 'Would you feel comfortable having a conversation with someone who didn't make eye contact?' Unfortunately, many of the findings make for sober reading. In 2024 the issues the community face feel altogether too similar to those that my family and I encountered in the late 1990s. The struggle to get into school, the battle to get professionals to understand, the lack of meaningful inclusion in the local community being but a few small examples.

We have all heard the adage that 'The more things change, the more they remain the same.' In Ireland, things have undoubtedly changed greatly in a relatively short space of time in terms of views and attitudes towards autism. Yet the decision-making and societal expectations that have caused our community such hurt often seem to repeat themselves. We have battled for years to ask people to not just become aware of us but to understand and accept us. And perhaps, in the true spirit of the United Nations Convention on the Rights of Persons with Disabilities, it is time we ask non-autistic people to become self-aware of their attitudes and the steps they can take to remove barriers for our community.

Priyangee Guha is a lawyer, celebrant and comedian. She is a firm believer of 'No such thing as too much cake.' In their spare time you will find her crocheting and watching the same TV show for the 73rd time.

Radical Love

Once upon a time I decided to relocate to a new continent where I knew no one. It was by no means an impulsive decision. I don't make impulsive decisions. Even trivial decisions like which foot I use to take the first step are well thought out. You may not see the reasoning, but it is there – like faith or love or Covid. I was in the depths of my anxiety and burnout (which I would learn a year later was autistic burnout). I was keen on a fresh start. I wanted to reset, restructure and re-imagine my life. And I did restart – just not the way I had envisioned. Fate read my memo, and instead of doing as I said, decided to give it a *creative* spin.

The year was 2020. I was *fresh off the boat* to Ireland. I moved here with 35kg of possessions packed in two suitcases, 70kg of anxiety packed in one brain and a licence to practise law, which I could not use in this country. What could possibly go wrong? I was trying to make sense of things with my therapist. I had been working with them for a few years. We started our sessions trying to help me process secondary trauma as a result of working with victims of violence. That gradually progressed to other topics. One such conversation has stayed with me.

It was a crisp winter morning, unusual for that time of the year with all four seasons in one day. It was sunny, windy and cold simultaneously. I grabbed a cup of tea, covered myself with my fuzzy blanket and turned on my laptop.

Skype pinged with my therapist saying they were ready for the session. We have been doing Skype sessions from the beginning – only audio, no video, thank heavens for that. We were very ahead of our time, I suppose. We were scheduled to discuss the assessment we had done prior to the session – Ritvo Autism and Asperger Diagnostic Scale (RAADS), and Aspie Quiz. While I did not understand the technical aspects of the assessments, I knew what the result could be. I have been dealing with my central processing unit for my entire life, after all.

'The results show that you are autistic,' they said after going through the assessment form in detail.

I responded with my trademark monotone 'OK.'

'How do you feel about it?'

'Nothing really. It is like someone saying, "You are diabetic." It is what it is, and it is good to know because now I can take steps to mitigate harm and plan life incorporating this identity. Am I supposed to feel different?'

Years later I would learn that my response was an anomaly. People have all kinds of responses to the assessment initially – fear, anger, depression, sadness, joy. For me, it was as straightforward as saying that the earth is round. I have been working with the disability community as a lawyer and policy expert for years. I learnt self-acceptance, love and kindness from them. Of course, we all bounce around a little about how we feel about ourselves, but that is only natural, isn't it? I embraced my identity as autistic. I controlled my urge to deep-dive into the subject. By then I also knew to steer clear of write-ups by 'experts', family members of autistic people and anything that was written from the lens of deficiencies. I delved deeper into my life – as much as a chronically depressed brain allowed – and suddenly things began to make sense. I found the root cause of my strengths and weaknesses: autism. I found the root cause of my abilities and disabilities: autism. I found the root cause of my differences and indifferences: autism. I found Me.

What next? I tried to go through the Rolodex in my brain to see if I knew any autistic persons: none. Then I expanded the search: did I know *of* any autistic person? I did: Hannah Gadsby, world-famous comedian from Australia. *That's it. I'll sign up for stand-up*, I told myself. I opened the search engine, researched for open-mic opportunities for beginners and signed up for a gig. Turns out, unbeknown to myself, I have been writing the script for a long time. Ever since I was a little girl I have had no shortage of people in my life mocking me. At some point, after I turned twelve, I realised that I had to take control of the situation. So I started mocking myself before I could be mocked: self-deprecating humour. Using comedy, I flipped the narrative.

Now, I dare you to find a country that enjoys self-deprecating humour more than Ireland. I fit right in. I used my stage time to talk about being a disabled immigrant in a new country – intersectional representation, they called it. At every gig, at least one person would tell me that they felt seen and heard. My aim here was not to get a Netflix special. My aim was simple: one day, someone will look through *their* Rolodex to see if they know any autistic persons – either for themselves or for someone they love. They will find a name. The Rolodex will not be empty. It will at least have *my* name.

Yes, a new identity in a new place helped. But Ireland is culturally extremely hard to navigate for someone who did not grow up here and is also autistic. Allow me to elaborate. I tend to take things literally – 'a couple of minutes' means two minutes, 'yer man' means my partner, and it took me a long time to realise that when someone called me a 'gas cunt' they were not discussing my flatulence frequency. But in Ireland, people rarely say what they mean, or mean what they say. 'Grand, so' could be anything from being ecstatic to being mortified to being angry. I have rarely heard people say 'No.' Everyone asks 'How are you?' but never pauses even for a second to get a response. Small talk, especially about the weather, is taken as seriously as GAA and rugby. But Ireland is also a place with a slightly better understanding of autism than India. Most people know someone in their immediate circle who is autistic. In India, it is usually 'my brother's colleague's neighbour's cousin's son, or Sheldon Cooper'. Sure, this may not translate to adequate infrastructure. But compared to where I come from, it is significantly better. It's all relative, isn't it?

The newness of my life in Ireland and my life as an (aware) autistic person overlapped. I could tell people I was autistic here from day one. This came in very handy. You'd be surprised by the number of people who knew me prior to my assessment who point-blank refused to believe it. Apparently I masked so convincingly that they could not believe I was autistic. If you know someone on the Oscars committee, maybe you should give them my details for nomination? Anyway, I did not have to go through that here. I had a choice to make – to mask, like I did in India, or to be radically visible. I chose the latter.

At this point, let me pause and talk about radical visibility. There is a common misconception about radical visibility. Some think that people are talking about their marginalised identities (gender, sexuality, race, disability and so on) to seek attention. While that may be the case for some (I cannot be the spokesperson for every self-advocate in the world), it could not be further from reality. In fact, me talking about being autistic is strongly detrimental to me in every conceivable way. I may be refused employment, or medical treatment, or legal rights, or dates, or friendships. I have to educate every professional I meet about autism and specific needs that I have – doctors, nurses, trainers, interior designers. Additionally, I had to rebuild boundaries with friends and family. I lost a few of them in the process.

People who are self-advocates rarely do it for their own benefit. They are acutely aware that they may never see the changes they advocate for. That is not how public policy works. I would have said public policy moves at glacial speed, but global warming is going to prove me wrong. So, I will say: it moves slower than glacial speed. Yet, the self-advocates plough on because they do not want the next generations to go through the same struggles that they had to endure. They do it because they hope when a young child who just found out they are autistic opens a search engine and types 'autistic Indian' they will get several search results, and they will know that there is more to autism than how deficient they are. The decision of being a self-advocate and being radically visible is: Radical Love, for you and yours.

Mike McGrath-Bryan is a well-meaning young fella from North Cork. His main preoccupation over the years has been features-writing, including for the *Irish Examiner* and *The Echo*. He's currently trying lots of other new things, but is afraid of jinxing any of them.

Dordán (Drone)

Life is full of music. It's everywhere. I hear it in the world around me, where my partner and I live now, on Cork city's working-class northside. I can't imagine a world without it; from childhood wonder and the tumult of adolescence; to parsing our lives, identities and understandings in adulthood. It's in my blood – my dad played bass, inspired by the early influence of fellow Crumlin man Phil Lynott; my mam sang the O'Riada Mass as part of her school choir for Raidió Éireann in a church in Doneraile, Co. Cork.

I discern rhythm and melody in the world around me. Swelling from the evening hum of nearby roads up to Mayfield and Montenotte; escaping long-form from the gaping maws of gulls that cruise inland to shelter from the rain and stuttered out by starlings that line the trees of Glen Valley Park like crotchets and quavers; the irregular rhythms of a dripping kitchen tap that hasn't quite been turned off yet, or the faint whispers of electricity, audible from the walls, as devices and televisions and other distractions cool down after a day's utility.

I'm autistic, and an ADHDer. The 'ha'penny place' between the need for calm and routine to regulate, on one hand; and the urge for novelty and action to be kept engaged, on the other. I was diagnosed with both autism and ADHD as an adult, and my own journey, mapping the various territories of mind, body and the liminal spaces between, is ongoing.

Wired Our Own Way

My childhood and adolescence were spent mainly between the towns and villages that lie along the N20 between Cork and Limerick, where life revolves in large part around the drone created by liminality itself. The radios, tape-decks and televisions in our childhood homes carried word of a wider world; pictures and sounds that reached out, words and sentences invested with ever more fascinating meaning, imagery and feeling, which brought warmth to cold days and added miles to indefinite summers on an earth vibrating under our feet.

Our father's bass rig loomed large in our home, while our mother's love of art and creation formed our early influences. My favourite childhood book was *Silas Rat*, a revenge tale propelled forward by the rabid pen of illustrator Tim Booth, the name of whose old band in the book's biography raised even further curiosity: Dr Strangely Strange?

My brain chemistry was irreparably altered by glances of Northern rockers Therapy? as *The Den* signed off for the evening, the video for the single 'Nowhere' etching itself into my subconscious, a kaleidoscopic visual effect warping and distorting singer and guitarist Andy Cairns, sporting a bob-and-goatee combo, as he wielded a Gibson SG.

The big wide world of music accessible to a rural child ricocheted between the popular musical waves of the time, but there the idea – of connection, of closer-to-home – would lie dormant. Music wasn't just the wallpaper of the daily grind, nor a mute, static thing, solely to be admired from afar.

★

Along came adolescence. The big feelings, new awarenesses, unwritten rules, the swings and roundabouts of being utterly lost, within and without, for no real reason, glass barriers becoming more apparent.

Life seemed to come naturally to some, and I couldn't help but watch, grow fearful of inadequacy; dwelling on anxiety and inability to act, passed moments and missed connections. I couldn't muster the courage to ask a girl out, but I could channel the paranoia to ask one of the lads if he was really my friend.

The pale green glow of a cheap stereo in a darkened bedroom as I hunkered down and belatedly interrogated the name and sounds of Nirvana via their eponymous 'hits' compilation. The goosebumps that became discernible by how the light played on them, as 'Lithium' told me, and me alone, about what was, what could be. I felt invincible.

I wore band T-shirts like armour, rifled through magazines, spent computer class looking up band websites. I couldn't understand why others didn't see what I saw, hear what I heard, feel what I felt coursing – through batteries on my Discman, through the music, through my ears – into my brain.

Childhood's passing musical names reappeared on shop playlists, sending me bolting to the A–Z shelves of CDs; while hints of this whole other sonic world being closer than I thought unveiled themselves in the present, with names like Giveamanakick and Ten Past Seven, in bargain bins, second-hand racks and small shops I had to muster that certain courage to walk through the door of.

I set about picking up instruments because I wanted a piece of that feeling, whether from mystique-fuelled vainglory or the simple pursuit of an outlet. I had the intention, but the playing didn't quite come together for me the way it seemed to do for others, either in terms of practice or inspiration. I could see all the moving parts, but they disappeared when they were in my hands.

But at the same time I was also making friendships that would mean the entire world, and I could escape into them. I felt seen, heard, and in turn I listened back, let down my defences and had arguments, and things dawned on me differently.

Emails, and texts, and meetups where I could suddenly stand to make eye contact. We even thought we were cool when we decided to make each other mixtapes, parallel conversations, connections unfurling and unfolding at our own pace, hopes as high as our dander amid a future we barely knew how we'd get to, at a time when promise was everywhere.

Then the phone rang, and the world stopped.

A band T-shirt, handed to an undertaker to go atop a friend's coffin. Eyes that used to widen at the mention of music now looking up from the pages of a newspaper. The days, weeks and months that followed fell into an endless grey and, as social and economic doors slammed shut after a failed Leaving Cert, the colour began to drain from my vision as bright futures and high hopes retreated behind veils of uncertainty.

For a few years I sleepwalked through life. I booked small gigs and promoted them, trying to do a service to a local scene whose potential was, to me, writ large. Building a platform, I told myself, in my delusions of grandeur. I wore the vogueish clothes of a noughties music blogger, filling my days with the humdrum of hobbyist media admin, and my nights with gig-going.

That drone emerged from the earth again, this time from a local noise collective I'd booked as emergency openers for a melodic metal band. Low hums, textures drifting in and out, broken up with squalls of warbly guitar that weren't quite atonal, but certainly not of any familiar world. No barriers here, nor the dreaded block of things to learn, internalise and reprocess. I instinctively asked if I could join the collective after their set.

They put up with me for about a year of empty bars and full arts-centre halls, of slow learning and elusive signs of 'progress' before I was summarily informed by one lad that another thought I was 'a bit much'. I had somehow been thrown out of an improvised noise ensemble.

Notions of new-media dominance, avant-garde tomfoolery and events-management glory gave way to finding ways and means of making things work. After years of begging-bowl emails, a last-minute interview with Blindboy Boatclub of the Rubberbandits led to a regular place in Cork newspaper *The Echo*, where I not only learnt how to adapt my interest-driven communication style for a broader readership in a way that was creatively satisfying, but also how to strike various balances and lend an established platform to local makers, doers and dreamers.

My enthusiasm was met and, in that desire to help, slowly but surely, connections, common causes and good friendships came together.

The pandemic brought life to a standstill. For those of us fortunate enough to still be working, it did not quite represent an escape from the pace of normal life but signposted a change in the balance of work, life and systemic navigation.

Diagnosis was dispensed remotely, with the kindness and empathy we all needed amid the distance and anxiety. Suddenly, here was context, here was understanding. Not excuse, but explanation – a connection lost in the shuffle of life, survival and the chase for whatever higher ground presented itself.

Unpacking old anxieties and hurts, new perspectives on events, relationships and traumas, bawling to a friend in the back of a pub, it hit me that I had lost touch with that intrepid young fella and his desire, however ill-informed, to start a punk band. Learning to convey my needs, realising that it was OK to start something new from scratch, and to ask for time and grace to make mistakes and learn.

Coming away from Culture Night at the Kabin in Hollyhill with the bare tools of traditional guitar accompaniment, spurred on once more by the earth's drone as it was coming to a generation through the bodies and voices of avant-trad explorers Lankum, mending the post-colonial, late-capitalism heart by bridging the innate with the possible. Offering practical contributions alongside rediscovered enthusiasm, in exchange for patience, I started to move past old fears, exclusions and heartaches.

Sharing a stage with Liam Ó Maonlaí. Helping with a beginner's trad session in our city's library. Breaking long-standing, heavy silences with old friends, and tending to those wounds together. Making peace with the limits that met frustrated aspirations. Talking with others in a similar place, about their own moves past hurt and into the present – sharing, bonding, connecting.

Dusting off old dreams and placing them with due care alongside new ones.

When I go home, and my mam and I talk about Seán Ó Riada, her mind invariably turns to that formative experience of the radio, the excitement of being heard, of her and her classmates' voices being carried along the airwaves and around the country. Without missing a beat, she shares the music and words, never forgotten, always present, a legacy handed down to her in a country still forming an idea of itself, and to her children's generation in their own turn.

I attended the Leeside launch of his son Peadar Ó Riada's book, charting the work and legacy of the legendary Ceoltóirí Chualann, modernisers and keepers of the living tradition. Music for the Ó Riada family and their musical peers has been a tether, a root, to our land, ourselves, our cultural inheritances and the factors that birthed them.

Peadar spoke of childhood memories of his father's work, the company he kept, and became tearful at the recollection of family members playing and dancing in the kitchen. The intangible, the moment, the everlasting, the cherished. Inextricable from the love, the passion and the drive inherent to the music.

It was hard to fight the tears that came when I tried to thank Peadar for preserving the legacy and work that had given my mother the same power.

Those connections, that sense of place, that sense of time, that agency – resonates for a lifetime, following us all along and down into an earth that drones along for another generation.

Aisling Walsh is an award-winning writer with work published in *The Guardian*, *The Irish Times*, *Jezebel*, *Electric Literature*, *Literary Hub* and others. She received an Arts & Disability Connect grant in 2023 and an Irish Writers Centre bursary in 2024.

Ticklish Brain

Deep in the abyss I feel someone hitting me. I hear voices, distant, but getting louder. I want them to shut up. It's nice down here, in the dark, away from my body, away from the world. It's peaceful and I'm ever so tired.

Why do they have to ruin it by dragging me back to the surface? I resist a few minutes more but the voices from beyond become ever more insistent. A crack in my eyelid floods my vision with light. I blink a couple of times and, as my eyes come into focus, I see six nurses standing over me, all wringing hands and furrowed brows.

I don't understand what they are doing nor why I'm on the floor. My tongue traces a newly jagged edge of my front tooth. I pat my nose, searching for my glasses, but all my fingers find is raw skin. Wet and heavy cotton clings to my thighs. I close my eyes and wish once more for the abyss.

This was the third seizure of only seven that I have had in my whole life. The first one happened when I was eighteen; the last one happened six months ago. The seizure described above, which earned me a diagnosis of epilepsy, just happened to take place at Cork University Hospital (CUH) while I was accompanying my mother to the out-patient's clinic for a post-op check-up. I was twenty-three and on my summer holidays between the second and third year of my degree. When the nurse removed the bandage from my mother's wound, the knot in my stomach turned to nausea and a cold sweat broke out on my forehead. I made it as far as the chair and heard ringing in my ears just before the darkness descended.

These sensations have become a familiar warning sign, not just of a likely seizure, but that my body has reached its limit of physical and emotional stress. A seizure is like a shutdown and reboot on a computer that has frozen or is overheating. The injuries and public incontinence can be very upsetting, not to mention the repercussions for driving and other activities. Still, the profound rest and sense of renewal that follows a seizure, the excuse to switch off and do nothing for a few days, can be an incomparable relief. After fifteen years of mapping the pattern of seizures to personal crises, I have figured out that a seizure is a way of my body telling me 'enough is enough' when I have failed to identify or heed other signs of fatigue, burnout or crisis.

The neurologist who diagnosed me with epilepsy after a two-minute consultation had no interest in interrogating the history nor the circumstances of my seizures. He did not seem to think it relevant that when I had the seizure in CUH my mother was terminally ill with cervical cancer and I was supposed to be learning how to take care of her colostomy bag following the latest, and final, palliative intervention. He did not consider the possibility that, after a year of watching my mother fade away in front of my eyes, neither my brain nor my body could handle more stress.

The witness account of the nurse who saw me go down trumped any explanation I might have had. He said simply: 'Your brain reacts differently to stimuli than most people's. It's more sensitive, ticklish if you will.'

★

In hindsight, he was not altogether wrong. But my brain is ticklish in ways I could not fully comprehend until I was diagnosed with autism, three years ago.

Like many women, as well as queer, trans, nonbinary people and people of colour, my autism had been missed or misdiagnosed (bad behaviour, insolence, rebelliousness, depression, anxiety) by parents, teachers and therapists alike. I spent most of my adult life believing I was broken and seeking out intensive therapy aimed at 'fixing' myself and my emotional problems. At thirty-seven, floundering through yet another relationship and friendship crisis so similar to those which had come before, I began to wonder if maybe something else was going on.

Articles about late-diagnosed autistic and ADHD women kept finding their way to me. The more I read the more I felt as if these women had entered my subconscious and laid bare the secrets about myself I guarded most closely: the disconnect with other people, the difficulties making and sustaining friendships and relationships, the deep need for silence and alone time so long ignored, the sensory sensitivities, the stop–start attempts at pursuing a career (or multiple attempts at different careers), the persistent imposter syndrome, the recurring burnouts and the sense that things were getting harder despite the years of therapy.

After months of reading and research, accompanied by an increasingly intense dialogue with myself about whether I could be neurodivergent and what that would mean, I decided to seek an assessment. I knew that without the external validation I would never fully trust my own perception of myself, nor feel legitimate about assuming any label. The outcome of the multiple questionnaires, screening tests and interviews I took all confirmed that my experience of the world did, in fact, align with autism. I thought diagnosis would be the end of the journey, but it was only the beginning.

As I began to read and understand autism and neurodivergence, I realised that my experience is characterised, among other things, by extremely sensitive sensory perceptions and nervous system. At the same time, I learnt about the interoceptive sense and realised that I experience significant difficulties in identifying emotions and bodily sensations. Somehow I knew that the key to understanding my seizures lay in the interaction between my ticklish brain and my difficulties in recognising and regulating emotional and physical overstimulation.

As a child and teenager I externalised all the anger and frustration of navigating the often incomprehensible and overwhelming world of neurotypical expectations in rages that shook the walls of my home. My mother and brothers bore the brunt of my internal chaos. It became clear that the consequences of these meltdowns could be disastrous for me – my mother issued an eviction notice at eighteen, just two weeks after the Leaving Cert. She could no longer tolerate me at home and apparently was at a loss for alternative solutions. I was left on the doorstep with two suitcases that I hauled between friends' houses for the summer as I looked for a job and somewhere to rent. It was such a shock that I turned the rage inwards. I focused all my energy on letting none of my distress show on the outside, on hiding the monster lurking inside me from the world, determined to avoid repeating that kind of rejection.

It was that year my seizures began. All seven seizures I have experienced have been preceded by some kind of emotional upheaval or physical pain. Sometimes they happen in the moment of crisis, sometimes there is a delay.

With a little time, a lot of distance and a mutual desire to find another way to relate to each other, my mother and I eventually made our peace. The day I accompanied her to the hospital the armour of false confidence, of a daughter who thought she was handling her mother's terminal prognosis, crumbled. My mother's wound, the undeniable advance of her illness, the level of care it would require and the knowledge that the time we had to rebuild our relationship would be brutally cut short could no longer be denied. It was just too much to handle. My brain short-circuited and then hit reset. I suspect the seizure was a moment of autistic shutdown, not the first but certainly the most public, and possibly the most spectacular, of all my seizures. But even as my body screamed for help, nobody, least of all me, knew how to interpret what had happened.

While researching an essay on trauma for my PhD I fell down an internet rabbit hole on dissociation. At the bottom of that hole, in a far corner of the internet, I found a link explaining how dissociative disorders can lead to seizures, which look and feel like epilepsy but are not neurological in origin. I realised that the disconnect I often feel between the body and mind could be connected to the habit of dissociation learned after decades of accumulated trauma and the interoceptive difficulties that are a common feature of autism.

I have since learnt that autistic people are 7 per cent more likely than the general population to have epilepsy and up to 20 per cent of people who have regular seizures may be experiencing non-epileptic seizures. Epilepsy medication does nothing to treat nor prevent dissociative seizures. Rather, specialists recommend therapy, early diagnosis and support in dealing with psychological disorders, distress and neurodivergence. Without subjecting myself to more testing, I can never say with 100 per cent certainty whether my seizures are a symptom of epilepsy or not. Nor can I speak for the experience of other people in the wider autistic community or others with epilepsy. But I feel, in my gut, that my seizures are a product of the autistic see-saw between meltdowns and shutdown, where a shutdown, even one as serious as a seizure, remains the more socially acceptable expression of overstimulation.

I never got to explain any of this to my mother. She passed away within a month of my epilepsy diagnosis. She was forty-seven, I was twenty-three. The origin of my seizures, the deep trauma of growing up with undiagnosed autism and the impact that our misunderstandings over my neurology had on our relationship are just some of the many conversations we never got to have. I often wonder what she would make of me now: about to hit forty and only just beginning to understand the complexities of my ticklish brain.

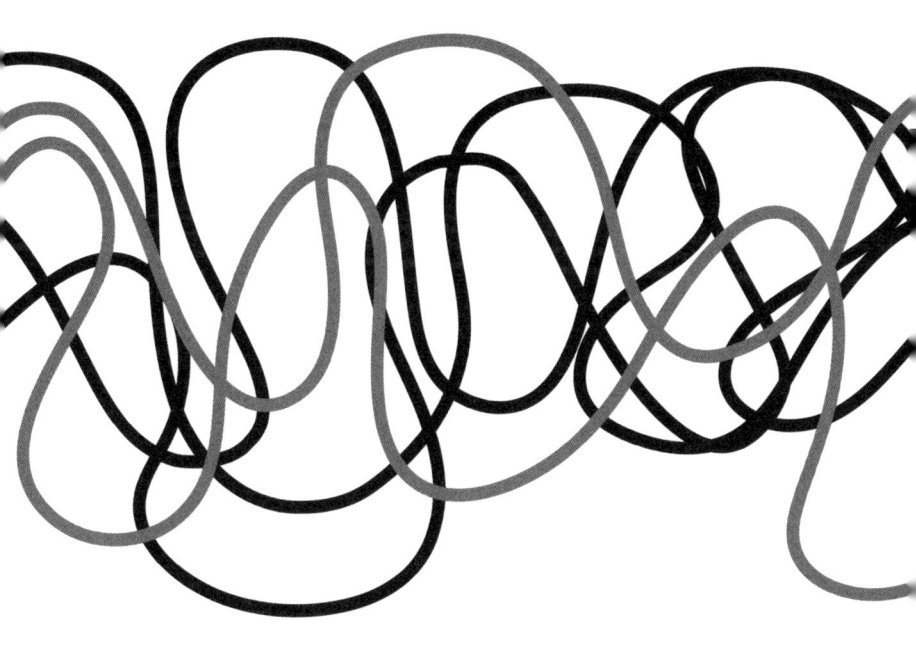

Cliona Kelliher works in the climate field and received a MSc in Climate change in 2022, as well as a diagnosis of autism. She writes a blog about her life experiences, including autism, at **puritybelle.com**. She is presently studying autism in UCC.

The Magic of Books

Books and reading have been a thread that has interwoven every part of my life, since I was very small.

I read early and incessantly, devouring books like they were life's sustenance itself. I read beyond the level for my age and focused on fiction mainly, although in later life academic studies brought me into other spheres.

My memories of childhood are fuzzy and grey, with little pictures occasionally emerging from the fog, but a consistent theme is that I remember books and stories – not just the narrative but also how they made me feel and think about life beyond my own little world.

I read all the Enid Blyton books as a child, loving the adventure and mystery of the *Famous Five* and the *Secret Seven* – which led to a lifelong interest in mystery and detective fiction. *The Faraway Tree* tales opened a window to magical kingdoms and strange creatures.

The Little House on the Prairie series engrossed me completely; I could almost feel the cool water of the creek and smell the smoke of the stove. I didn't just read about Laura, I *was* Laura, just as I was Jo from *Little Women*. In the absence of social acceptance, I was mirroring and learning to mask, but I was also creating a world in my head where I would be liked and would fit in, be brave and kind and adventurous.

I was very much a little girl and adolescent who was on her own. Yet I'm not sure that I felt lonely. Perhaps at times

I did, but certainly in those periods when I was on my own with a book, I had no sense of loneliness. I became part of the story. It was as real to me, possibly even more real, than the physical world around me.

Books influenced my sense of self, my vocabulary and how I express myself verbally. They have contributed to my strong sense of justice and my intense dislike of unfairness. Books were my reality. They parented and guided me. Marmee in *Little Women* was how I wanted everyone to be – she understood each of her daughters, who were all so different, and gave each of them what they needed to blossom and feel loved.

The 'out there' territory of real people and real social situations was jarring by comparison. I didn't have friends in real life due to my social awkwardness and extreme shyness. Book characters were easier to befriend; they behaved in ways that were predictable.

Apart from the Enid Blyton mystery books, another story that I loved was *The Murders in the Rue Morgue* by Edgar Allan Poe. Interestingly, this has been described as the first modern detective story and it introduced me to the Gothic mystery genre, full of intrigue and set amidst foggy streets, with strange conundrums that I figured out alongside the protagonist. Sherlock Holmes, Hercule Poirot and Walter Hartright were my friends for a while and they led to a whole world of crime and mystery fiction where being immersed in a puzzle gave me endless joy; to this day, this is my favourite way to switch off and decompress for a while.

Moreover, it wasn't just the reading of the books that I relished, it was also the physicality of books. There is something really nice about the weight of a book and the rhythm of turning the pages, that little swish sound as your fingers move and your eyes seek out the next word.

I often read on my iPad now but when I was younger, any bookshop was an immediate draw for me, particularly if they had old books. I've always been quite sensory-seeking, enjoying touch and nice smells, and that old-book smell is incredibly evocative for me, allowing endless imaginative potential. Books with personal inscriptions were an added bonus – there is something so lovely about diving into a book that someone long ago also read. I could imagine them sitting in an armchair, by a fire perhaps, and reading the same lines that I was reading. It gave me a glimpse into connections that were missing in my own life.

If I visit your house, any bookshelf will pull me like a magnet and I'll want to explore the titles and read the synopses. It takes quite a bit of restraint for me not to engross myself immediately in the reading material; books won't make me feel awkward or worried about saying the wrong thing.

I've kept a collection of books, mainly hanging on to those that hold special memories or classics that I really enjoyed and will often reread if I have nothing else to read. Dickens, Trollope, the Brontës and Jane Austen are all authors whose books I have picked up many times. And that rereading is often a comfort for me if I'm feeling dysregulated – the familiarity is soothing in the same way that I find comfort in re-watching all the *Star Trek*s.

In terms of non-fiction, doing my master's introduced me to the more scientific world of academic papers and books. Although I can't speed-read through these at quite the same pace I use for reading fiction, being exposed to this type of literature opened up new windows in my head and I discovered that I absolutely loved absorbing swathes of information that would engage every part of my brain. I developed confidence in my own opinions and began to understand that having a different perspective wasn't necessarily a bad thing, was often positive in fact.

It was during pursuit of my master's that I got my autism diagnosis and began learning all sorts of new terms and concepts related to neurodivergence. Understanding that a lot of my struggles were integral to my autism and not some inherent flaw, while also being able to celebrate that some autistic traits brought me joy and benefit, was a healing road for me. When I learnt about the term hyperfocus, it described so perfectly my feeling of intense total absorption, a feeling that was both pleasurable and calming. It was like everything in my head just shifted into perfect alignment for that brief period. And of course, the love of researching and getting all the detail on a topic is something many autistic people relate to. This was of huge benefit to me in the academic arena, and acknowledging that was part of a long process of learning to accept myself.

Many autistic traits are framed as deficits and it's infrequent that we hear more positive words like joy. However, special or focused interests can be a huge source of joy. It's so clear to me now that books were one of my earliest special interests, and a central interest that has endured throughout my whole life. Not only that but books have led me down many other paths, meandering away, returning and developing. From books came my love of language and the intricacies of linguistic expression, as well as communication in general. I'm fascinated by the sounds of words and how they magically flow together to express feeling and atmosphere. How someone else's crafting of a phrase can bring sense and meaning to our own emotions and experiences. I still love the feel of books and the comfort they evoke in me. They feel like a little oasis to me where I can dive into another universe and forget about myself for a while.

In the somewhat topsy-turvy world I experienced post-diagnosis, where I questioned everything about myself, I began to understand that reading and books were an integral part of the real me, the uncamouflaged core of who I was. Like a little kernel of reality that I could build on, and allow to grow. Like a story that's just beginning, yet has always been here in the lore of humanity.

Timeline of Autism Diagnosis: An Overview

1911 The first recorded use of the term 'autism' was by psychiatrist Paul Eugene Bleuler, developed from the Greek word *autos* for 'self'. Bleuler used the word 'autism' to reflect the symptoms of social withdrawal and self-absorption, which he had identified in a cohort of people with a diagnosis of schizophrenia.

Early 1900s Autistic children (or at least the ones with traits obvious enough to get a diagnosis) would have been labelled with either 'childhood schizophrenia' or 'mental retardation'.

1925 Grunya Sukhareva, a child psychiatrist, published a paper on what she called 'schizoid personality disorder', which is now widely thought to be the first paper identifying a group of autistic children. She later changed the label to 'autistic psychopathy'.

1940s Scientific papers were published by child psychiatrist Leo Kanner (in the US) and paediatrician Hans Asperger (in Austria) describing children who had a collection of behaviours that included communication differences, social withdrawal and intense interests. Despite not being aware of each other's work, Kanner labelled this subset of

1960s

'symptoms' as 'early infantile autism', while Asperger labelled it as 'autistic psychopathy'. A psychologist named Bruno Bettelheim (along with Leo Kanner) claimed that autism was caused by cold and unloving mothers, whom he called 'refrigerator mothers'. Despite this theory being disproven, it enhanced the shame and stigma around autism.

In America Dr Ole Ivar Lovaas founded Applied Behaviour Analysis (ABA), which was – and still is – a widespread education method that aimed to reduce undesirable behaviour (i.e. autistic behaviour) and promote socially typical behaviour in autistic children. He also played a prominent role in the creation of 'conversion therapy' as a 'treatment' for gay and transgender people. Both these 'therapies' grew from the concept that one's authentic identity could and should be suppressed to fit in with social norms.

1970s

Lorna Wing, a UK psychiatrist, conceptualised that autism was a spectrum. She identified that there are many ways to be autistic, and that all autistic people do not fit into the typical male presentation of autism as previously thought. This led to a huge jump in the amount of people recognised to be on the 'autism spectrum'.

1980s

The American Diagnostic and Statistical Manual of Mental Disorders (known as the *DSM*) separated the labels of autism from the umbrella term of 'schizo phrenia'. Autistic children were now diagnosed with 'infantile autism' instead of schizophrenia.

1990s The *DSM* and the World Health Organization's International Classification of Diseases (the ICD) split the label of autism into 'Asperger's syndrome' for people with no speech delay and 'autism disorder' for those with speech delay, and often those deemed to have below average intelligence.

2013-2019 Both the *DSM* and the World Health Organization's ICD removed the diagnostic label 'Asperger's syndrome' and all other autism-related labels (included PDD-NOS, classic autism, Rett syndrome and so on) and now use the umbrella diagnosis 'autism spectrum disorder' or ASD for all people identified as autistic.

Present time The rise of autistic adult voices sharing their experience of autism has led to an increased understanding of the lived experience of autism, which has led to an increase in autism identification. This is fuelled by the ability to connect with other autistic people via the internet, autistic people carrying out and publishing neuro-affirmative (rather than deficit-based) research into autism, and a change in how autism is assessed and recognised, for example the inclusion of sensory processing differences as part of an autism assessment.

A Note on Language around Autism

The language around autism has changed in recent years. Previously, professionals tended to encourage people to use 'person-first' language and say that a person 'has autism' rather than 'is autistic'. This was thought to be more respectful, by allowing people to separate themselves from a medicalised diagnosis. Nowadays, autism is no longer seen as a medical condition, but is recognised as a natural and normal neurotype (albeit one that can be very disabling, particularly when the environment is not designed for their autistic needs).

The majority of autistic people have called for 'identity-first' language, in recognition that our autism is an intrinsic part of us, and not something detachable. We therefore say we are 'autistic' rather than that we 'have autism'. I use this identity-first language in this book, but some writers use different language. The language people choose to use about themselves can be a very personal thing, and I asked the writers to use their own preferences when talking about themselves.

Glossary

AAC (augmentative and alternative communication): This is any communication method used instead of speech, or alongside speech, to enhance communication efficacy. There are multiple types of AAC, from writing to flash cards to using technology to text, type or generate speech. An AAC device refers to a device or app that generates speech when the user taps or types the words they wish to communicate.

AAC user: This refers to someone who uses an AAC device to communicate.

ADHD (attention deficit hyperactivity disorder): ADHD has many different presentations, from difficulties with attention and focus to hyperactivity and impulsivity. Research has shown that 40–70 per cent of autistic people have ADHD.

Alexithymia: A difficulty or inability to recognise and name one's emotions.

AsIAm: Ireland's national autism charity.

Aspie: A shortened name for the now outdated diagnosis of Asperger's syndrome. Asperger's syndrome now falls under the general diagnosis of 'autism spectrum disorder'.

Autistic burnout: A period of reduced quality of life with chronic exhaustion, stress and increased sensory sensitivities, which occurs when the expectations and demands placed on an autistic person outweigh their ability to fulfil them. To be considered true autistic burnout, this period tends to last for three months or more.

Hyperfixation: An intense interest or preoccupation with something that takes up a lot of the autistic person's time and/or thoughts.

Masking: Hiding to hide one's autistic traits. Autistic people usually begin masking to protect themselves from stigma, ridicule, or bullying. By adulthood, masking can be so ingrained as a self-protective measure that autistic people are not always aware when they are masking. It can therefore be conscious or subconscious.

Meltdown: An emotional 'explosion' that occurs when an autistic person becomes suddenly overwhelmed, or when overwhelm builds up over time and eventually hits boiling point. Like non-autistic people, when an autistic person's nervous system responds to extreme stress, we experience 'fight, flight or freeze' mode; a meltdown is autistic 'fight' mode. Not all autistic people experience meltdown; some will respond to stress with 'flight' or 'freeze' (also known as an autistic shutdown). Autistic meltdowns present in many different ways, including uncontrollable crying, shouting, running away, shaking, curling up in a ball and physically releasing stress.

Montropism: A person with a monotropic mind tends to focus very intently on something of interest, and may not take information in from anything else around them. They may also find themselves constantly thinking about their topic of interest, even when not engaged in it.

Glossary

Neurodiversity: Similar to how 'biodiversity' refers to the diversity of life in nature, neurodiversity refers to the diversity of the types of brains (neurotypes) that are natural to humanity. This includes both neurotypical and neurodivergent brains.

Neurodivergent: A neurodivergent person has one or more different neurotypes to a neurotypical person. Examples of neurotypes that are considered neurodivergent include autistic, ADHD, OCD, dyslexic, dyspraxic and Tourette's.

Neurotypical: A person who has a 'typical' brain, i.e. is not neurodivergent.

Shutdown: While a meltdown is an external 'explosion' of emotion due to overwhelm, a shutdown is an implosion of emotions that manifests as a person 'shutting down'. This can present as an inability to communicate, socially interact or carry out tasks. It is temporary and tends to pass within a few minutes, hours or days, when the autistic person's nervous system calms down.

Stimming: Engaging in a repetitive behaviour to self-soothe or regulate oneself, especially when feeling intense emotions. Examples of stims include physical movement such as hand-flapping, twirling hair, spinning, rocking, spinning a ring on a finger; making repetitive sounds with one's voice, including humming, singing a tune repeatedly, saying words over and over; counting, thinking the same words again and again, like a poem or prayer; or banging, tapping, listening to the same song on repeat.

Voice-generating app (aka speech-generating app): This is a type of AAC. The user of the app chooses what they want to communicate, and the app generates speech, i.e. says what the person wants to communicate out loud. The user can input their message into the app using whichever method suits them, whether that is through typing words into the app, tapping images or words, using eye-gaze technology or pressing buttons (knowns as switches).

Acknowledgements

An anthology is, by its very nature, created by multiple people. This is quite the opposite to my usual experience of writing books, which can be quite solitary. It has been a wonderful experience to bring people together to create this beautiful record of Irish autistic lives, and I am so grateful to everyone who played a role in its creation.

I wish to extend a huge thank you to Mariel Deegan and Djinn von Noorden from New Island Books for being such a wonderful team to work with. They brought so much enthusiasm and insight to this book, and I will miss our many chats and discussions about autism and the essays. I also wish to thank Des Doyle for his role in the promotion of the book, along with everyone at New Island Books who was involved in this project.

I relied on many other people to get the word out about this anthology, which is how I managed to get as diverse a range of writers as possible. Thank you to all the organisations and people who helped to distribute my call-out for essays, with a particular thanks to Elske Rahill, and Ireland's national autism charity AsIAm.

In the end, I collected an abundance of essays, many of which didn't end up in the anthology. It was a hard choice to pick the ones that worked best together as part of a collection, and I am very grateful to all the people who submitted essays and shared their experiences with me. Thank you to Stefanie

Preissner for kindly allowing us to reprint her essay which first appeared in the *Irish Independent*.

An enormous thanks to the Arts Council for supporting this book. Thank you for giving autistic Irish adults the chance to have their real-life stories cemented in printed text.

Thank you to Nina, who alerted me to the fact that Mariel Deegan had posted a message on Facebook explaining her interest in publishing a book on the topic of autism. And finally, a heart-felt thank you to my family, especially my husband Cathal who celebrated and supported my work on this book from the beginning to the end.